THE
GUIDE
PRESCRIPTION
DRUGS

THE
GUIDE TO
PRESCRIPTION
DRUGS

DR MARK GOYEN

Michael O'Mara Books Limited

For Sandy and Julia

This edition published in 1996 by Michael O'Mara Books Limited
9 Lion Yard, Tremadoc Road
London SW4 7NQ

First published in 1991 by The Watermark Press Sydney

Copyright © Mark Goyen 1991, 1994, 1996

Revised 1996

Text adapted by Henry Morriss BSc Hons

A CIP catalogue record for this book is available from the British Library.

ISBN 1-85479-718-2

Printed and bound by Cox & Wyman, Reading

Foreword

The range of drugs available today is staggering. The development, manufacturing and supply of therapeutic drugs is a multi-billion dollar world-wide industry. Even for a doctor, the task of keeping up to date in pharmacology is daunting. In medical school, emphasis is given to cover even the more common drugs in great depth in the time available. Thus keeping up to date with drugs is an ongoing process for all doctors. From the patient's perspective it is a little more straightforward. Most patients on drug treatment receive a small number of medications at any one time. Thus it is possible, with a little time and research, to 'get to know' the drugs you are taking.

Modern drugs can be dramatically effective. For example, 20 years ago, many operations were performed for ulcers of the stomach and duodenum. Today, due to the development of drugs that decrease acid production by the stomach, these operations are relatively rare.

One point cannot be over emphasised. One doctor, usually your GP, should be aware of all the medications you are taking. It is surprising how many people continuously 'shop around' for medical care. While identifying a good doctor to whom you can relate is clearly important, it is equally important to have a doctor who has an in depth knowledge of your problems and is coordinating your treatment. There are many examples of drugs that interact and may be dangerous when combined with certain other drugs. Equally, certain drugs that may be safe for most patients, may be extremely dangerous in the presence of certain medical conditions. An accurate knowledge of the drugs you are taking, have been taking in the past, and your medical condition, is essential for good prescribing by your doctor.

This guide provides basic and easy to read information regarding a range of more commonly used drugs. Use it to understand the drugs with which you are being treated. Also, it should encourage you to ask your doctor more specific questions concerning the likely benefits and side effects of your treatment. As always, being an informed consumer is in your best interest.

Dr Christopher Liddle
Department of Clinical Pharmacology
Westmead Hospital, Sydney

Introduction

The most recognisable aspect of modern medicine is the prescription of medications. To some extent our culture encourages us to accept a cure with a pill as being the identifiable solution to a definable problem. Yet it has not always been so, and it may not be so in the future.

It is important therefore to stress, that pharmacological cures for illness are only one of many possible solutions. I emphasise this point as it can easily be lost in a book which deals exclusively with medications, almost all of which must be prescribed by a medical practitioner.

Even so, I have always felt that there is a definite requirement for a straightforward consumer guide to prescription medicines, especially those which are most commonly used. Each entry in this guide is designed to be read as a whole. While the brevity of the text accentuates the important points, the idea is to read from the top to the bottom and get a 'feel', or general understanding of a drug and how it works.

Medical jargon must be the most confusing language on earth. For people with medical backgrounds it makes communication precise and avoids misunderstandings. But when used between doctor and patient, medical jargon is often confusing. For this reason I have gone to some lengths to make the book simple. The central concept is that it should be possible to hold the book open with one hand, and the prescribed medication in the other. Hopefully, this will allow the consumer to get the relevant information about each drug without having to refer to other medical texts.

Each entry should be seen as a summary of a summary of a summary of the sum total of information known about each drug. The information selected for inclusion has the average consumer in mind and attempts only to include those points which are pertinent.

This leads me to the most important point of the introduction. The GUIDE TO PRESCRIPTION DRUGS is not designed to be a textbook, but merely the briefest introduction to 230 or so of the most commonly prescribed medications today. I can't emphasise more strongly that any queries you may have about a particular medication should be discussed with your doctor. Even a comprehensive textbook on pharmacology will probably not give the quality of information that you need about a medication and how it will affect you.

Also, as a result of the strict editing process that has reduced a mountain of information down to a brief discussion of each medication, it is clear that some people may develop problems with particular medications that are not even mentioned in the book. While I apologise for this, I must make it clear that omissions are unavoidable in producing a popular yet concise guide.

In this new edition there are 30 additions to the drugs described and only 3 deletions. These new additions are far from exhaustive. Many of the drugs are so-called 'designer drugs', purpose built molecules which owe much to a more fundamental understanding of the biochemistry of the body and the ingenuity of the scientists who 'tailor make' a drug. These drugs are quite exciting trend setters and naturally their development comes at a price.

Also of interest is the trend of making drugs easier to use. There has been an explosion of the development of once a day medications, by altering drug molecules, by slowing the absorption of the tablet in the gut and by the innovative use of skin patches to allow absorption through the skin. Again this trend will continue, and lead to a vast improvement in patient compliance and convenience.

Dr Mark Goyen
August 1994

A word on the correct use of drugs

There is little doubt that the proper use of medicines can be of great benefit in healing a wide variety of illnesses. However, misuse can be tragic, and all too often it is completely unnecessary. Of all the drug-related poisoning cases reported by hospitals most are the consequence of accident rather than abuse. Many could have been prevented by following a few simple rules. Before you use any medication, please take the time to read this list of precautions.

DO become familiar with the exact effects of your medication. Talk over potential effects and side-effects with your doctor.

DO be careful to follow the instructions on your medication.

DO talk to your doctor about possible alternatives to medication. Remember all medications affect the body. There may be a better way.

DO be sure to keep your doctor(s) informed of all your prescriptions. As you will see in this book, many drugs interact with others, sometimes in ways that are very dangerous.

DO consult your pharmacist about over-the-counter medication. These may also interact with other drugs.

DO ask your doctor or pharmacist what precautions, if any, should be taken when using medication. For example, alcohol often has an adverse reaction with other drugs.

DON'T share prescribed medications with anyone else. Similarly, don't use anybody else's prescribed medication. Different drugs have different effects on different people, even if the symptoms are the same.

DON'T keep old medicines lying around the house, especially if they have passed their expiry date. These drugs, if taken, may have unexpected results.

DON'T allow children access to medicines. For their sakes, and yours, make sure all medications are kept well out of their reach.

* The advice above has been drawn from an advertisement published by the Pharmaceutical Benefits Scheme, a Commonwealth Government Health Care Program.

acyclovir

Trade Names	Zovirax
How Available	tablet, ointment
Drug Group	Anti-viral antibiotic
Prescription	Yes
Major Uses	This drug is used for treating viral infections caused by herpes viruses. It is useful for infections in the eye, around the mouth and for genital herpes. It can also be used to treat shingles (caused by the Varicella virus), if treatment is started early.
How it Works	Acyclovir prevents the herpes viruses from growing. It acts within body cells.
Usual Dosage	Up to one or two grams per day may be needed. The ointment should be applied as prescribed by your doctor.
Common Side-Effects	Uncommon. Nausea and vomiting, headaches and dizziness are the most common.
Actions with other Drugs	Any drug which reduces the excretion of acyclovir in the kidney can increase its side-effects. Probenecid is the most likely drug to do this.
Pregnancy, Breastfeeding	There is no known risk in either pregnancy or breastfeeding with topical use of acyclovir, but there is not enough evidence to determine if this is true if the drug is taken orally. Thus the oral medication is not recommended for use in pregnancy or breastfeeding.

alclometasone

Trade Names	Not yet available in the UK
How Available	cream, ointment
Drug Group	Topical Cortico-steroid
Prescription	No
Major Uses	This medication is used to treat many conditions of an inflammatory, but not infective, nature in the skin.
How it Works	Topical cortico-steroid preparations are effective in the treatment of many skin conditions because of their anti-inflammatory and anti-itch properties and because of their ability to constrict blood vessels. However, the exact way in which the drug works is essentially unknown.
Usual Dosage	Apply to areas of affected skin three times per day.
Common Side-Effects	Burning, itch, redness, irritation and dryness are the commonest side-effects, though rare. Other skin problems may occur.
Actions with other Drugs	Nil of note.
Pregnancy, Breastfeeding	Short term use of this medication is generally deemed to be quite safe, however, as some of the steroid is absorbed through the skin and into the circulation, it should not be used in excessive amounts or for prolonged periods of time. Short-term use in breast-feeding women is regarded as being safe.

allopurinol

Trade Names	Caplenal, Cosuric, Hamarin, Rimapurinol, Zyloric
How Available	tablet
Drug Group	Drug used for gout. Xanthine oxidase inhibitor.
Prescription	Yes
Major Uses	Allopurinol is most commonly used in people with gout. It helps to reduce the number of attacks of gout and also reduces damage done to joints during an attack. It can also be used in the treatment of any condition in which there is an over-production of uric acid. This includes some tumours. It helps to reduce kidney stones.
How it Works	The drug acts on an enzyme preventing the formation of uric acid. As a result, there is a reduction in the level of uric acid in the blood.
Usual Dosage	Most adult patients need from 100 to 300mg per day, as a single daily dose.
Common Side-Effects	Not common. A skin rash is the most frequent complaint. Nausea is also quite common. Other problems are rare. It is possible to bring on an attack of gout if the dose changes (either increasing or decreasing). It is often necessary to use another medication at the time that the dose of allopurinol is changed in order to prevent gout.
Actions with other Drugs	Anti-coagulants, such as warfarin, can be interfered with, and should only be used at the same time under strict control. Some diuretics may reduce the effect of allopurinol. Long-term use of iron tablets with allopurinol is not advised.
Pregnancy, Breastfeeding	The drug has not been proven safe in either pregnancy or breastfeeding, though it would be quite unusual for women in child-bearing years to take it.
Special Features, Comments	Alcohol may increase the adverse effects of allopurinol.

alprazolam

Trade Names	Xanax
How Available	tablet
Drug Group	Benzodiazepine
Prescription	Yes
Major Uses	This drug is used for the short-term relief of anxiety and the treatment of conditions which lead to panic in people with depression. It is not known if use for greater than a few months is beneficial.
How it Works	The exact action of this drug and of other drugs in the benzodiazepine group is not known. It works on the central nervous system.
Usual Dosage	0.25 to 1.5mg per day.
Common Side-Effects	Due to its central nervous system effect, drowsiness is the most common side-effect. Also dizziness and unsteadiness are common. Less likely are forgetfulness and confusion as well as nausea. Side-effects are more frequent in elderly people.
Actions with other Drugs	Any medication which can cause sedation will add to the sedative side-effects of alprazolam and vice-versa. Sleep drugs, antihistamines, antidepressants, strong analgesics and major tranquillisers will have this additive effect as will alcohol.
Pregnancy, Breastfeeding	Alprazolam has not been proven safe to take in pregnancy or while breast feeding, and its use is advised against in this situation.
Special Features, Comments	As with other benzodiazepines, there is a potential for dependence with long term use of the medication. Also overdosage can occur. Excessive sleepiness and the inability to arouse a person who has access to alprazolam should lead to the suspicion of overdosage. Immediate medical attention should be sought. Alcohol should be avoided with alprazolam treatment. Also, its effects can become weaker over time. Care should be taken while driving or performing hazardous tasks while the drug is being taken.

amiodarone

Trade Names	Cordarone X
How Available	tablets, injection
Drug Group	Heart-rhythm drug
Prescription	Yes - should only be initiated in hospital
Major Uses	This medication is used for the treatment of heart rhythm disturbances originating both in the upper section of the heart (the atria), and the lower sections of the heart (the ventricles)
How it Works	Amiodarone works by prolonging the electrical conduction time of various tissues within the heart. This means that there is an increase in the amount of time between cycles of electrical excitation of these tissues, with a net damping down of electrical activity.
Usual Dosage	The usual dose is between 100mg and 200mg per day. When the medication is commenced it is often given in higher doses, either orally or intravenously.
Common Side-Effects	Amiodarone has a number of important side-effects. It may cause a reduction in blood pressure if introduced quickly, and it may cause heart arrhythmias as well as treat them. It may make heart failure worse. This medication may affect liver function and also function of the thyroid gland. Blood tests need to be taken before and during therapy. People on the medication may develop a rash when exposed to sunlight and may develop a slate-grey appearance to the skin. Changes to the eye may occur and the cornea at the front of the eye may develop deposits, which can affect vision in people on high doses of the drug. Various other side-effects can occur.
Actions with other Drugs	Many of the other drugs used in the treatment of heart rhythm disturbances can potentiate the effects of amiodarone. These include beta-blockers, calcium channel blockers and digoxin. It should be used with caution with any other heart rhythm drug as it may cause a new rhythm problem or substantially lower blood pressure. In addition, amiodarone potentiates the anticoagulant effect of warfarin and may alter the blood concentration of other drugs within the body.
Pregnancy, Breastfeeding	Amiodarone is not recommended for use in either pregnancy or breast feeding.

continued over page...

amiodarone continued

Special Features,
Comments

It is important to monitor blood pressure as well as signs of heart failure. Blood tests for liver function and thyroid function should be taken at regular intervals. Regular reviews by an eye doctor are important, in people who are taking a large dose of the drug.

amitriptyline

Trade Names	Domical, Elavil, Lentizol, Triptafen, Tryptizol
How Available	tablet
Drug Group	Tricyclic antidepressant
Prescription	Yes
Major Uses	Amitriptyline is most commonly used in the treatment of depression. It can be used long-term and elevates mood, increases activity, appetite and gives a sense of well-being. Due to its sedating effects it is used in situations where sleep disturbance accompanies depression. It is also useful in children for the treatment of enuresis (bed-wetting), where other causes have been excluded.
How it Works	The exact way in which amitriptyline acts is unknown. It is known that it inhibits the uptake of some chemicals around nerve endings, but the effect of this is uncertain.
Usual Dosage	Usual dosage for adults is 75mg per day. This can be increased up to 300mg per day. The dosage for the treatment of bed-wetting in children is much less, often 10mg at night or slightly more depending on the child's weight and age.
Common Side-Effects	Due to its action on the central nervous system, amitriptyline's most common side-effect is drowsiness. This is expected when treatment commences. Also, a group of side-effects, known as anti-cholinergic side-effects will occur to some degree. These include a dry mouth, blurring of vision, constipation and difficulty passing urine. If a person has heart, eye or urinary problems, these should be discussed with the doctor before prescribing.
Actions with other Drugs	Any medication which can cause sedation will add to the sedative side-effects of amitriptyline. Sleep drugs, antihistamines, antidepressants, strong analgesics and benzodiazepines will display this additive effect as will alcohol.
Pregnancy, Breastfeeding	Safe use in pregnancy and breastfeeding has not been established. There are theoretical reasons why this drug should not be used in either of these situations, so it is not recommended.
Special Features, Comments	Heavy smoking may interfere with the effectiveness of the drug.

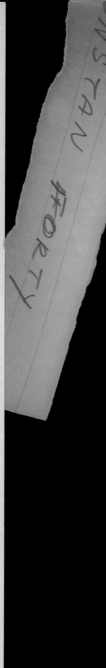

amlodipine

Trade Names	Istin
How Available	tablet
Drug Group	Calcium channel blocker
Prescription	Yes
Major Uses	Amlodipine is mainly used for the long-term treatment of raised blood pressure. In addition, it can be used in the treatment of angina.
How it Works	Calcium channel blockers are thought to work by preventing the influx of calcium ions into the cells of smooth muscle which line the walls of small arteries. This decreases blood pressure and also increases the flow of blood through arteries which may be partly blocked. It may also have some action in preventing spasm of the walls of partially blocked arteries.
Usual Dosage	2.5mg to 5mg once per day is the usual dose, though this may be increased to 10mg.
Common Side-Effects	Swelling of the feet, dizziness, flushing and palpitations are the commonest side-effects and these are related to the dose of the drug. These are commoner at the start of treatment. Many other side effects have been reported, but they are less likely.
Actions with other Drugs	Amlodipine enhances the effects of other medications which reduce blood pressure. However, there are no reports of other significant interactions with drugs. Interestingly, the level of amlodipine in the blood is increased when taken with grapefruit juice. This is thought to be due to a component unique to grapefruit, as it does not occur with other citrus fruits.
Pregnancy, Breastfeeding	Amlodipine should not be used in women who are pregnant or attempting to fall pregnant, as theoretically it has the potential to cause birth defects. It is generally not recommended in breast feeding.
Special Features, Comments	This medication should be used with caution in people with heart failure as it may make the problem worse. Alcohol may accentuate the blood pressure lowering effects of the drug.

amoxycillin

Trade Names	Amix, Almodan, Amoram, Amoxil, Amrit, Augmentin, Galenamox, Rimoxallin
How Available	tablet, capsule, syrup, injection
Drug Group	Penicillin antibiotic
Prescription	Yes
Major Uses	Amoxycillin is a widely prescribed antibiotic, which is active against a wide variety of bacteria. It is useful for the treatment of ear, nose and throat, urinary tract, respiratory tract, mouth and skin infections. It is also useful for the treatment of gonorrhoea. Augmentin acts on an even greater variety of bacteria.
How it Works	This drug works by stopping the growth of the cell wall of bacteria. It not only stops bacteria from growing, it also kills them.
Usual Dosage	This varies considerably from 500mg to 1.5g daily depending on the type of infection being treated, and other factors. In children, the dose is adjusted according to weight and age.
Common Side-Effects	A rash is the commonest side-effect of amoxycillin. (More severe allergic reactions are much less frequent. A severe rash or difficulty in breathing requires immediate medical assessment.) Nausea and vomiting as well as diarrhoea are the next most common side-effects. Vaginal thrush may be a possible problem in women. Nausea is perhaps more common with Augmentin.
Actions with other Drugs	Probenecid may increase the level of amoxycillin in the blood. Use of amoxycillin at the same time as the oral contraceptive pill may affect the absorption of the 'pill', and may compromise its contraceptive effect as well as possibly cause bleeding between periods.
Pregnancy, Breastfeeding	Amoxycillin has been taken by large numbers of pregnant and breastfeeding women. It has not been shown to have adverse effects on the unborn, nor breastfed babies. It is a commonly used antibiotic, if one is required in these situations.
Special Features, Comments	Overgrowth with fungus in the mouth and gastro-intestinal tract may occur with this medication if use is prolonged. The clavulinic acid component of Augmentin may sometimes cause liver inflammation.

amphotericin

Trade Names	Ambisome, Amphocil, Fungilin, Fungizone
How Available	lozenge, syrup
Drug Group	Antifungal antibiotic
Prescription	Yes
Major Uses	Amphotericin is used for the treatment of fungal infections in the mouth and around the teeth as well as the gastro-intestinal tract. It can be used to treat serious fungal infections throughout the body. Fungal infections in the skin can also be treated with this drug.
How it Works	Amphotericin causes damage to the cell membranes of funguses, thus destroying the cells.
Usual Dosage	Oral lozenges are low dose (40mg). The average oral dose for adults is 400-800mg per day.
Common Side-Effects	No side effects are usually reported with the lozenges or the oral tablets. Very rarely an irritation to the mouth may be due to use of the lozenges. Occasionally skin discolouration or a rash may occur with the topical preparation. If used for serious infections and given by vein, in hospital, many more side-effects are possible.
Actions with other Drugs	These do not occur with the oral tablets, lozenges, or ointment forms of amphotericin.
Pregnancy, Breastfeeding	There are no known risks with the oral tablets, lozenges, or ointment forms of amphotericin in either pregnancy or breastfeeding as it is not absorbed from the gastro-intestinal tract.

ampicillin

Trade Names	Amfipen, Ampiclox, Magnapen, Penbritin
How Available	tablet, capsule, syrup
Drug Group	Penicillin antibiotic
Prescription	Yes
Major Uses	Ampicillin is used against many bacteria for a variety of infections. These include respiratory tract, ear nose and throat, urinary tract and skin infections. It is similar to amoxycillin in its actions.
How it Works	Ampicillin prevents the cell wall of bacteria from being formed, thus destroying the bacteria.
Usual Dosage	250-500mg every six hours is the average adult dosage. Dosage in children is dependent on age, weight and the seriousness of the infection.
Common Side-Effects	Rash is the most common side-effect. (More severe allergic reactions are much less frequent. A severe rash or difficulty in breathing requires immediate medical assessment.) Nausea and vomiting as well as diarrhoea are the next most common side-effects. Others are rare.
Actions with other Drugs	Probenecid may increase the level of ampicillin in the blood.
Pregnancy, Breastfeeding	Ampicillin has been taken by large numbers of pregnant and breastfeeding women. It has not been shown to have adverse effects on the unborn, nor breastfed babies, and can be used if necessary.
Special Features, Comments	No substantial interaction with alcohol.

antazoline

Trade Names	Otrivine-Antistin
How Available	drops, ointment
Drug Group	Antihistamine
Prescription	No
Major Uses	This medication is used in combination with other local drugs in the treatment of allergic problems of the eyes, skin and nose as well as to reduce inflammation.
How it Works	Antihistamines prevent histamine from reacting with cells and causing local inflammation. [Histamine is a naturally occurring substance present in some white blood cells (mast cells)].
Usual Dosage	Apply to the affected area every three to four hours.
Common Side-Effects	These are uncommon. Local irritation or allergic inflammation may occur. Some combinations can lead to raised pressure in the eye. Other side-effects are possible if the combination medications are absorbed into the body.
Actions with other Drugs	Nil of note.
Pregnancy, Breastfeeding	These medications may be used in pregnancy and breastfeeding if necessary.
Special Features, Comments	The medications should not be used for prolonged periods without medical advice.

aspirin (acetylsalicylic acid)

Trade Names	Angettes, Aspirin, Caprin, Nu-seals aspirin
How Available	tablet, capsule, powders
Drug Group	Analgesic, anti pyretic, anti-inflammatory, anti-platelet aggregating drug
Prescription	No
Major Uses	Aspirin has been used for many years to relieve pain, reduce fever and inflammation. It has many uses from the treatment of simple headaches to menstrual pain, migraine headaches and severe inflammatory problems such as rheumatoid arthritis. More recently, it has been used in low doses to try and prevent strokes and heart attacks, by decreasing the clotting capacity of the blood.
How it Works	Aspirin blocks the function of an enzyme, cyclo-oxygenase which is important for the formation of substances known as prostaglandins. Some prostaglandins cause inflammation, some cause fever. Others are necessary for the normal function of platelets in the blood. (Platelets are responsible for one type of clotting in the blood.) Thus aspirin has a wide ranging number of actions on the prostaglandins in the body, actions which also lead to some side-effects.
Usual Dosage	Low doses (75-300mg per day) are all that are required to decrease the aggregating capacity of platelets. 300-900mg every four to six hours is necessary to reduce fever, pain and inflammation. Larger doses may be needed for acute rheumatic disorders. Aspirin is not recommended for use by children less than twelve years of age unless absolutely necessary (as in rheumatoid arthritis). It is also not recommended for children or teenagers suffering influenza, chicken pox or fever due to the possibility of a very serious, though rare condition, Reye's syndrome.
Common Side-Effects	Nausea and indigestion are common side-effects with aspirin treatment. Peptic ulcers and bleeding may occur. Anaemia is possible, while at higher doses, ringing in the ears may result. Severe allergic reactions can occur with aspirin, even with low doses which occurs in some foods. Damage to the kidneys and liver are rare, but possible problems.

continued over page...

aspirin continued

Actions with other Drugs

Other anti-inflammatory drugs, corticosteroids and alcohol will increase the stomach irritation caused by aspirin. Aspirin may interfere with anticoagulant drugs treatment. Some drugs used for gout prevention will be adversely affected by aspirin. Aspirin may increase the effects of drugs used for diabetes.

Pregnancy, Breastfeeding

Aspirin is not recommended for use in pregnancy or breastfeeding. In pregnancy it may prolong labour. In breastfeeding the drug is passed onto the baby and allergic problems may arise.

Special Features, Comments

Aspirin should not be used in people with a history of peptic ulcers, liver or kidney disease or bleeding problems. Alcohol could increase the inflammation of the stomach that aspirin causes. Aspirin may also impair the breakdown of alcohol in the stomach. Due to the blood clotting effects of aspirin, it should be stopped before surgery or dental work. Aspirin does not treat the cause of pain or inflammation and, if symptoms have not resolved within two days, medical advice should be sought.

astemizole

Trade Names	Hismanal
How Available	tablet, syrup
Drug Group	Antihistamine (non-sedating)
Prescription	Yes

Major Uses

Astemizole is used to dampen down allergic reactions. It is used for the treatment of hay fever (allergic rhinitis) and allergic conjunctivitis..It can also be used to treat longer term skin allergies.

How it Works

Antihistamines prevent histamine from reacting with cells and causing local inflammation. [Histamine is a naturally occurring substance present in some white blood cells (mast cells)]. Unlike many antihistamines, astemizole does not cross over into the central nervous system, and thus does not usually cause drowsiness, in the doses normally prescribed. It is long-acting and need only be taken once per day.

Usual Dosage

Adults usually take 10mg per day, while children take 2.5-5mg per day.

Common Side-Effects

Side-effects are uncommon with astemizole. It may increase appetite and body weight if used for a prolonged period.

Actions with other Drugs

The blood levels of some antihistamines can be increased with the use of erythromycin, which theoretically could cause a dangerous cardiac rhythm problem.

Pregnancy, Breastfeeding

Astemizole is not recommended for women who are pregnant or attempting to fall pregnant, though no definite problems with astemizole therapy have been established. Likewise, it is not recommended for breastfeeding mothers.

Special Features, Comments

There is no specific interaction with alcohol, unlike other antihistamines. Moderation of alcohol is, however, advised. Overdose should be reported as soon as possible as heart rhythm disturbances are possible.

atenolol

Trade Names	Antipressan, Tenoret 50C, Tenormin
How Available	tablet
Drug Group	Beta-blocker
Prescription	Yes
Major Uses	Atenolol is most commonly used to treat raised blood pressure. It also may be used to treat angina (pain from an inadequate oxygen supply to the heart). It is sometimes used after a heart attack to prevent further damage to the heart muscle. Some disturbances of heart rhythm may also be treated by atenolol.
How it Works	The means by which atenolol decreases blood pressure is not known. It decreases heart rate, and this is one of the reasons it is effective in angina, but this does not explain its ability to lower blood pressure. It has a direct effect on an area of the heart responsible for the rate at which the heart beats, controlling some rhythm disturbances.
Usual Dosage	50-100mg daily is the usual adult dose for blood pressure control.
Common Side-Effects	Muscle aches and pains are the most common. Cold hands and feet and general tiredness are possible. Sleep disturbances and nightmares can occur as can impotence. Rashes can occur, but are rare. If blood pressure falls too much dizziness is possible, especially on standing.
Actions with other Drugs	Antacids may interfere with the absorption of atenolol. Verapamil may accentuate atenolol's rhythm slowing and blood pressure lowering effects.
Pregnancy, Breastfeeding	Atenolol has been used for the treatment of raised blood pressure in pregnant women without recognised adverse effects. It can lower the fetal heart rate, which may be important at the time of delivery. It is not suggested for use by nursing mothers.
Special Features, Comments	It can be dangerous to withdraw this drug suddenly. People with diseased arteries to the legs may have worse symptoms. Unstable diabetic patients should avoid atenolol as it may mask low blood glucose levels. People with asthma or chronic bronchitis should avoid atenolol. It may make their problems considerably worse. The drug may need to be stopped before a general anaesthetic is given. An overdose of this medication can be serious and immediate medical attention should be sought.

auranofin

Trade Names	Ridaura
How Available	tablet
Drug Group	Anti-inflammatory drug (rheumatoid arthritis)
Prescription	Yes
Major Uses	Auranofin is a form of a salt of the metal gold, which can be given orally. It is of use in the treatment of rheumatoid arthritis, and not for other types of arthritis. It usually takes some months for an effect to be noticed. Other anti-inflammatory treatment is usually given at the same time.
How it Works	Auranofin has a wide range of effects on the immune system, though the exact way that it acts in rheumatoid arthritis is not known.
Usual Dosage	6mg per day is the usual adult dose, though this may be slightly higher. The medication is usually taken for a period of some months before response can be assessed. Auranofin is not recommended for use in children.
Common Side-Effects	Diarrhoea, nausea, vomiting, abdominal pain, flatulence, a rash, itch, sore tongue, mouth ulcers and inflamed eyes are all common with this drug. Other less common problems do occur. The most serious of these is a decrease in formation of blood cells and an inflammation in the kidney.
Actions with other Drugs	Other anti-inflammatory drugs may increase the chance of kidney inflammation with auranofin.
Pregnancy, Breastfeeding	This medication is not recommended for use in pregnancy or breastfeeding. Women wishing to become pregnant should stop the medication for six months before the intended pregnancy.
Special Features, Comments	Blood and urine tests must be performed at regular intervals to ensure that any severe side-effects are detected as soon as possible.

azatadine

Trade Names	Optimine
How Available	tablet, syrup
Drug Group	Antihistamine
Prescription	No
Major Uses	Azatadine is used to relieve allergic reactions. It is used for the treatment of hay fever (allergic rhinitis) and allergic conjunctivitis. It can also be used to treat more serious allergic problems and widespread allergic problems.
How it Works	This drug is a long acting antihistamine. Antihistamines prevent histamine from reacting with cells and causing local inflammation. [Histamine is a naturally occurring substance present in some white blood cells (mast cells)]. Azatadine also prevents the release of histamine.
Usual Dosage	The usual adult dose is 1mg twice per day for adults and 0.5-1.0mg twice per day for children.
Common Side-Effects	Drowsiness is the commonest side-effect. Numerous other effects have been recorded but are rare.
Actions with other Drugs	Any medication which can cause sedation will add to the sedative side-effects of azatadine and vice-versa. Sleep drugs, antidepressants, strong analgesics and benzodiazepines will display this additive effect.
Pregnancy, Breastfeeding	This medication is not recommended for pregnancy or breastfeeding, though definite harm has not been established.
Special Features, Comments	Alcohol adds to the sedative effect of this drug. People driving or involved in hazardous work should be aware of the possible sedative side-effects of azatadine.

bacitracin

Trade Names	Cicatrin, Polyfax, Tribiotic
How Available	ointment, cream
Drug Group	Topical antibiotic
Prescription	Yes
Major Uses	Bacitracin is used, often in combination with other antibiotics, to treat local infections in the skin. It is also sometimes used for external ear infections. Due to its toxic nature it cannot be used orally.
How it Works	This medication inhibits bacterial cell wall synthesis.
Usual Dosage	Topical ointment.
Common Side-Effects	Local allergic reactions are relatively common with one or more of the components of these topical antibiotic combinations.
Actions with other Drugs	As the drug is not absorbed, no interactions occur.
Pregnancy, Breastfeeding	It is important for nursing mothers not to use these preparations near the nipple or breast to prevent accidental ingestion by the baby.

beclomethasone

Trade Names	Aerobec, Beclazone, Becloforte, Becodisks, Becotide, Filair Forte inhalers, Propaderm
How Available	inhaler, nasal spray, aqueous nasal spray
Drug Group	Corticosteroid
Prescription	Yes
Major Uses	Beclomethasone is the sole active constituent of the above products. It is used to control the symptoms of allergic rhinitis (hay fever) in the nasal spray form. When used via an inhaler, it helps reduce the number of and severity of asthma attacks. It must be used before the attack of asthma occurs in order to be effective and the full effect of the drug may only be achieved after one or two weeks treatment.
How it Works	This medication is a very active anti-inflammatory drug. The drug works directly on the tissues in the lung and nose preventing inflammation. The exact way that it does this is not well understood.
Usual Dosage	2-4 puffs of the inhaler or the nasal spray 2-4 times per day depending on the severity of the disease. (The dose in different strength inhalers varies from 50 to 250 micrograms per puff.)
Common Side-Effects	No serious side-effects are likely with either form of this drug. Little of the drug is absorbed and the danger of it causing side-effects due to absorption into the body is low. Most commonly experienced with the inhaler are a dry cough and sore throat. Nose bleeds can occur with the nasal spray but nasal stuffiness and congestion are more likely.
Actions with other Drugs	No interactions are expected.
Pregnancy, Breastfeeding	There are no known problems in using this drug during pregnancy or breastfeeding.

bendrofluazide

Trade Names	Aprinox, Berkozide, Centyl-K, Corgaretic, Inderetic (with propranolol), Inderex (with propranolol), Neo-Naclex, Neo-Naclex-K, Prestim
How Available	tablet
Drug Group	Thiazide diuretic
Prescription	Yes
Major Uses	The major use of bendrofluazide and this group of drugs in general is the treatment of high blood pressure. It can also be used to reduce fluid build up in women prior to menstrual periods. It also reduces fluid retained in diseases of the heart, liver and kidneys.
How it Works	This drug works in the kidney to decrease the reabsorption of salts and water.
Usual Dosage	2.5-10mg daily dependent on indication.
Common Side-Effects	Leg cramps can occur. Prolonged use can lead to a depletion of potassium. Often a potassium replacement is used at the same time to prevent this potential problem.
Actions with other Drugs	Thiazide diuretics may make digitalis a more dangerous medication to take, because of the possible depletion of potassium. Lithium levels in the blood may be affected.
Pregnancy, Breastfeeding	In some situations in pregnancy this drug may be dangerous, and thiazide diuretics are not used. It may cause a reduction of blood flow to the fetus. Milk supply may diminish when it is used by breastfeeding mothers, so it is not commonly used.
Special Features, Comments	Long-term treatment may impair glucose tolerance, mimicking diabetes, though stopping the drug reverses this. An increase in uric acid level may be caused and possibly lead to gout. In severe liver disease this medication may be dangerous. The hangover effect of dehydration from alcohol may be made worse by bendrofluazide. Blood tests may be necessary from time to time to check on potassium levels. Thiazide diuretics may alter blood cholesterol levels.

benzocaine

Trade Names	Intralgin, Merocaine, Rinstead Adult Gel, Tyrozets
How Available	lozenge, liquid, syrup, other topical preparations
Drug Group	Local anaesthetic
Prescription	No
Major Uses	Benzocaine is commonly used to numb inflamed or painful tissue. While it is effective in relieving local symptoms, it does not alleviate the cause of inflammation, which may need to be treated separately.
How it Works	Local anaesthetics temporarily interfere with the transmission of impulses along nerve fibres. In low doses, they are most sensitive on the fibres responsible for pain sensation.
Usual Dosage	As per proprietary information.
Common Side-Effects	Reactions to the medication are rare, but skin reactions can well occur. Other allergic reactions are less common. In such situations use of the medication should be discontinued and further advice sought.
Actions with other Drugs	Nil known.
Pregnancy, Breastfeeding	As the medication is not absorbed into the body, there is no specific problem likely with benzocaine alone.

benzoyl peroxide

Trade Names	Acetoxyl, Acnecide, Acnegel, Acnidazil, Benoxyl, Benzagel, Nericur, Panoxyl preparations, Quinoderm (with hydrocortisone), Quinoped
How Available	lotion, ointment
Drug Group	Anti-acne drug
Prescription	No
Major Uses	Helps to reduce acne.
How it Works	Benzoyl peroxide stops a bacterium from breaking down sebum (a type of fat) in the skin to fatty acids which irritate the skin, thus causing inflammation and acne. It also helps to dry the skin.
Usual Dosage	Apply one to two times per day.
Common Side-Effects	Local irritation is a common side effect of this drug, as is drying and peeling of the skin. These effects are more common in people not used to the medication and if higher concentrations of the drug are used. Burning or stinging in the skin is a common sensation also. If this persists, then the preparation should be stopped.
Actions with other Drugs	Sometimes use with a sunscreen may lead to skin discolouration. Any cosmetic or other medication which dries the skin may add to the drying and irritating effect of benzoyl peroxide.
Pregnancy, Breastfeeding	There is no evidence of problems.
Special Features, Comments	This medication should not be used for more than a few weeks without medical advice.

benztropine

Trade Names	Cogentin
How Available	tablet, injection
Drug Group	Drug for Parkinson's disease
Prescription	Yes
Major Uses	Benztropine is used in the treatment of Parkinson's disease (a disorder of movement). It is very useful in treating the tremor and stiffness of the disease. It can also be used to treat movement problems, which result from the use of major tranquillisers.
How it Works	This medication blocks the part of the nervous system known as the cholinergic nervous system and also acts as an antihistamine.
Usual Dosage	0.5mg to 6mg per day is the usual adult dose for maintenance treatment. It is not recommended for use in children.
Common Side-Effects	Rapid heart rate, drowsiness, dry mouth, sweating, dizziness, blurred vision, constipation and difficulty passing urine are common side-effects with this medication and relate to the way in which the drug acts.
Actions with other Drugs	All drugs, including alcohol which have a sedative effect will have an additive effect on benztropine. Sleep drugs, antihistamines, other antidepressants, strong analgesics, benzodiazepines and major tranquillisers are the most common examples. If used with phenothiazines any abdominal bloating or discomfort should be reported as soon as possible.
Pregnancy, Breastfeeding	Although no specific problems have been proven, it is not recommended that benztropine is given in pregnancy or breastfeeding unless absolutely necessary.
Special Features, Comments	An overdose of this medication can lead to serious consequences. Confusion, excessive drowsiness, unconsciousness and exaggerated side-effects should suggest the possibility of overdosage. Immediate medical care is essential. Regular eye checks are necessary, as this medication may lead to increased eye pressure (glaucoma). Due to its sedative properties, it is important not to drive or do dangerous work until the effect of the benztropine on the individual is established. Alcohol will increase sedation.

benzydamine

Trade Names	Difflam
How Available	mouth gargle, ointment
Drug Group	Anti-inflammatory analgesic
Prescription	No
Major Uses	This drug is used as a locally active anti-inflammatory agent. It is effective for painful mouth and throat conditions as well as tonsillitis. It is used for local inflammation of skin, soft tissues and joints.
How it Works	It prevents the formation of chemicals which are responsible for local inflammation. (These chemicals are called prostaglandins.)
Usual Dosage	15ml as a gargle as needed. Applied to areas of inflammation as needed.
Common Side-Effects	These are rare. The mouthwash commonly causes numbness which may help relieve discomfort. Occasional burning and stinging in the mouth is also possible. If swallowed, nausea and vomiting may be caused.
Actions with other Drugs	Nil known.
Pregnancy, Breastfeeding	This drug is not recommended for use in pregnancy or breastfeeding, though there is no definite evidence of ill effects.

betahistine

Trade Names	Serc
How Available	tablet
Drug Group	Histamine-like drug
Prescription	Yes
Major Uses	This is most commonly prescribed for problems of the inner ear. These include dizziness and vertigo, Merniere's disease (a specific disease of the inner ear) and ringing in the ears (tinnitus) .
How it Works	This drug acts like the naturally occurring drug, histamine. It acts on histamine receptors on various cells of the body and may improve blood supply to the inner ear.
Usual Dosage	Up to 8mg 3-4 times daily.
Common Side-Effects	Nausea, vomiting, headache and dizziness are the most common effects.
Actions with other Drugs	Antihistamines decrease the effect of betahistine.
Pregnancy, Breastfeeding	This medication is not recommended. Safety in pregnancy and breastfeeding has not been established.

betamethasone

Trade Names	Betnelan, Betnesol, Betnovate, Diprosone, Fucibet, Lotriderm
How Available	tablet, cream, ointment, other topical preparations
Drug Group	Corticosteroid
Prescription	Yes
Major Uses	Most commonly betamethasone is used on the skin to treat conditions caused by inflammation and allergy. It can also be taken by mouth in situations where insufficient adrenal hormones are produced or increased amounts of hormones are necessary.
How it Works	This medication relieves inflammation in the skin. In oral form it increases the amount of cortisol in the blood stream.
Usual Dosage	Applied to skin as prescribed.
Common Side-Effects	In treatment of skin problems for short periods problems are rare. Long-term treatment, however, can lead to thinning of the skin. Local allergies to the preparations are also possible. There are many potential problems which may occur if betamethasone is taken orally. (See prenisolone/prednisone)
Actions with other Drugs	There are no likely interactions with the topical medications. (For interactions of the oral drug, see prednisone)
Pregnancy, Breastfeeding	Topical preparations do not present any problems. In low doses the oral tablets are unlikely to cause problems, but this should be discussed with your doctor.
Special Features, Comments	(See prenisolone/prednisone)

bromazepam

Trade Names	Lexotan
How Available	tablet
Drug Group	Benzodiazepine
Prescription	Yes
Major Uses	Bromazepam is used for the short-term treatment of anxiety, tension and agitation.
How it Works	The exact action of this drug and of other drugs in the benzodiazepine group is not known. It works on the central nervous system.
Usual Dosage	3mg 2-3 times per day.
Common Side-Effects	Most side-effects are accentuations of the nervous system actions of bromazepam. Drowsiness, unsteady walking and dizziness are the most common, while behaviour, sleep and speech problems are less frequent.
Actions with other Drugs	Any medication which can cause sedation will add to the sedative side-effects of bromazepam and vice-versa. Sleep drugs, antihistamines, antidepressants, strong analgesics and major tranquillisers will display this additive effect as will alcohol. In people who are epileptic, it may be necessary to increase the dose of some anticonvulsant medications in order to prevent an increase in seizure numbers.
Pregnancy, Breastfeeding	Bromazepam is not recommended for use in either pregnant women or breastfeeding mothers.
Special Features, Comments	People should be warned that bromazepam may impair mental skills, so that driving and dangerous occupations should be approached cautiously. This medication may cause withdrawal symptoms if removed from the system abruptly, and changes in dose should only be made on doctor's advice.

bromocriptine

Trade Names	Parlodel
How Available	tablet
Drug Group	Prolactin secretion inhibitor
Prescription	Yes
Major Uses	Most commonly, this drug is used to suppress breastfeeding in mothers who wish to stop. It is also used to decrease prolactin secretion, as well as growth hormone secretion (when it is increased as in acromegaly). Bromocriptine can also be used in the treatment of Parkinson's disease.
How it Works	This drug inhibits the release of prolactin and growth hormone from the pituitary gland at the base of the brain.
Usual Dosage	Breastfeeding suppression; 2.5mg twice daily for 14 days. Increased prolactin secretion; 1.25-2.5mg twice daily. Other conditions; doses are usually higher and depend on response.
Common Side-Effects	Confusion, nausea, dry mouth and dizziness are most common. In higher doses, and especially in people who use the medication for Parkinson's disease, hallucinations, confusion and other such problems may occur. Bleeding from the stomach is a serious, but rare side-effect.
Actions with other Drugs	Some anti-psychotic drugs may make Parkinson's disease symptoms worse, so may counteract the effects of bromocriptine. Metoclopramide may decrease bromocriptine's actions.
Pregnancy, Breastfeeding	As it may be used to treat some types of female infertility, many pregnant women have taken bromocriptine for some time in early pregnancy. No particular problems have been found, but it is still best to avoid this medication. Bromocriptine will suppress breast milk production completely if given just after birth.
Special Features, Comments	Due to its potential to cause drowsiness, driving and skilled work may be affected. Alcohol will increase confusion caused by the drug.

budesonide

Trade Names	Pulmicort, Rhinocort
How Available	turbohaler, inhaled aerosol, nebulising solution, nasal spray
Drug Group	Corticosteroid
Prescription	Yes
Major Uses	Budesonide is the active constituent of the above products. As a nasal spray, it can be used to control the symptoms of allergic rhinitis (hay fever). In inhaled form, it decreases the number and severity of attacks of asthma. It must be used before an attack of asthma occurs, and it may take a few weeks of regular usage for the complete effect of the medication to become apparent.
How it Works	This medication works very effectively as an anti-inflammatory agent in both the airways of the lung and the nasal passages. The drug acts on these tissues dampening down the inflammatory response of abnormal tissue. The exact way this occurs is not known, though one of the effects is to reduce the production of inflammatory mucus.
Usual Dosage	The usual dose is 2 to 8 puffs or inhalations per day. The actual dose of medication prescribed varies dramatically, as the puffers and turbohalers come in various strengths.
Common Side-Effects	Generally the medication is well tolerated. Little of the medication is absorbed into the body, and that which is, quickly becomes inactivated in the liver. Most side-effects are local reactions. Hoarseness, sore or irritated throat, dry mouth, cough and oral thrush are possible with the inhaled preparations. Nasal stuffiness or runny nose are possible as well with the nasal spray.
Actions with other Drugs	No significant interactions have been reported with budesonide.
Pregnancy, Breastfeeding	If the use of cortico-steroids is necessary for the control of asthma during pregnancy, then it is preferable to use an inhaled drug such as budesonide. Generally, it is not recommended that breast-feeding women use the drug.

bumetanide

Trade Names	Burinex
How Available	tablet
Drug Group	Loop diuretic (fluid tablet)
Prescription	Yes
Major Uses	Bumetanide is used to remove excess fluid from the body. This is necessary in heart, liver and kidney failure. It is also used to lower blood pressure, often combined with other medications.
How it Works	Bumetanide inhibits the kidney's ability to concentrate urine. The result is that the kidney produces a far greater quantity of urine.
Usual Dosage	1mg daily is the usual adult dose, though this may be increased considerably if necessary in severe kidney or heart failure. Bumetanide is usually not used in children below the age of eighteen years.
Common Side-Effects	Dizziness, nausea, headaches, muscle cramps and low blood pressure are the commonest side-effects with bumetanide treatment. Electrolyte disturbances are common biochemical abnormalities. The levels of potassium and sodium in the blood can be altered. Blood tests at regular intervals may be necessary. A rash can occur, though more serious allergic problems are unlikely. Many other side-effects are recognised, but are rare.
Actions with other Drugs	Some anti-inflammatory drugs can reduce the action of bumetanide. Other fluid tablets can accentuate the potassium losing properties of bumetanide. Toxic effects of digoxin are more common, if the blood potassium level is low. Some antibiotics and aspirin may cause hearing problems if given in high doses with bumetanide. Bumetanide may increase the level of lithium in the blood.
Pregnancy, Breastfeeding	It is possible that bumetanide may cause some problems in the fetus. It is not usually given and may adversely affect some women who have raised blood pressure in pregnancy. The medication may reduce milk supply. It does pass into breastmilk and is generally not recommended in breastfeeding.
Special Features, Comments	People with bladder problems may be adversely affected by the increase in urine production. Regular blood samples checking potassium levels may be necessary. Alcohol may lead to dehydration.

calcitriol

Trade Names	Calcijex, Rocaltrol
How Available	tablet
Drug Group	Vitamin
Prescription	Yes

Major Uses

This medication is most commonly used for the treatment of established osteoporosis, most commonly in women following the menopause. It can also be used in some cases of kidney failure and underproduction of parathyroid hormone, where bone density is affected. It can be used in Vitamin D deficiency.

How it Works

Rocaltrol is a form of Vitamin D which has undergone transformation from a relatively inactive form to the most active form. Vitamin D assists in the uptake of calcium from the small intestine and also the deposition of calcium in the bones.

Usual Dosage

This varies from the usual dose of 0.25mcg per day to 0.75mcg. Children also receive similar doses.

Common Side-Effects

Drowsiness, weakness, constipation and a raised blood calcium level are the commonest problems. The most worrying side-effects of the drug are due to excessive activity of Rocaltrol and thus increased serum calcium levels. In extreme cases, this may cause excessive thirst and urine production as well as weight loss.

Actions with other Drugs

Cholestyramine may affect the absorption of Rocaltrol. Antacids may cause a rise in the magnesium level in the blood. Thiazide diuretics may also elevate serum calcium levels.

Pregnancy, Breastfeeding

This medication is not recommended for use in pregnancy nor breastfeeding.

Special Features, Comments

It is important, that a track of serum calcium levels should be kept, with estimates of blood calcium levels taken, especially at the start of therapy.

captopril

Trade Names	Acepril, Capoten
How Available	tablet
Drug Group	ACE inhibitor (angiotensin-converting enzyme inhibitor)
Prescription	Yes
Major Uses	Captopril is used in the treatment of raised blood pressure and heart failure.
How it Works	Captopril works mainly by reducing the activity of the enzyme angiotensin converting enzyme to prevent the transformation of angiotensin I to angiotensin II. Angiotensin II is a very potent substance which leads to a marked increase in blood pressure, therefore, decreasing the levels of angiotensin II will lead to a reduction in blood pressure. A lowering in blood pressure can also reduce the workload of the heart and improve its function.
Usual Dosage	The drug is often started at a low dose and increased as tolerated. 12.5mg-150mg per day. This medication has not been proven safe for children and is not generally used.
Common Side-Effects	Dizziness and weakness can occur. An itchy rash is commonly experienced early in treatment, but usually disappears. A persistent, non-productive cough occurs in some patients. Nausea, vomiting, mouth ulcers and mouth inflammation may occur.
Actions with other Drugs	Some anti-inflammatory drugs may interfere with captopril's effectiveness. Diuretics (fluid tablets) may lead to an excessive fall in blood pressure, especially if captopril is not added slowly. This effect may also occur if other drugs which dilate arteries are used. Serum potassium levels may be raised by captopril if potassium sparing fluid tablets are used at the same time.
Pregnancy, Breastfeeding	This medication should not be used during pregnancy. Use of captopril is not recommended while breastfeeding.
Special Features, Comments	Captopril may worsen kidney function in people suffering from kidney disease. It may raise the level of potassium in the blood especially in people taking fluid tablets that spare potassium. From time to time, checks on blood chemistry should be made.

carbamazepine

Trade Names	Tegretol
How Available	tablet, liquid
Drug Group	Anticonvulsant (drug used for epilepsy)
Prescription	Yes
Major Uses	Carbamazepine is used for the treatment of a variety of fits. It is used as a long-term treatment to prevent fits from occurring. It is also used to treat some types of long-standing pain.
How it Works	This drug slows down or stops the transmission of some nerve endings in the brain.
Usual Dosage	Up to 2g per day in adults, though the usual dose is 400-600mg per day. Dosage in children depends on age, weight and response to treatment.
Common Side-Effects	Dizziness, tiredness, sedation and difficulty walking are seen when the drug is started. Nausea, vomiting and blurred vision are also possible. An itchy rash can occur.
Actions with other Drugs	Carbamazepine may interfere with the oral contraceptive pill (an increased hormone dose may be necessary), and with anti-coagulant treatment. Cimetidine may increase the effects of carbamazepine. The blood level of other drugs used for epilepsy may also be altered.
Pregnancy, Breastfeeding	Women who use anticonvulsant drugs during pregnancy do have an increased chance of having birth defects. The chance is about three times normal. In many cases, there is no alternative but to use anticonvulsants. The potential problems to mother and baby of uncontrolled fits during pregnancy outweigh the possibility of having an abnormal child. The drug is passed into breastmilk and safety in nursed infants has not been proven.
Special Features, Comments	Due to the sedative effects of the drug, driving and dangerous work should be undertaken with caution. Blood tests are usually taken to assess the level of carbamazepine in the blood. Alcohol can increase the sedative effect of the drug.

carbimazole

Trade Names	Neo-Mercazole
How Available	tablet
Drug Group	Drug for thyroid disease
Prescription	Yes
Major Uses	Carbimazole is used to suppress the thyroid gland in situations in which it is over-active. This most commonly occurs in a condition known as Graves' disease. Carbimazole can also be used to prepare the thyroid gland prior to surgery on the gland and also before other treatments to reduce the thyroid gland's activity. This medication may take some weeks to exert its full effect.
How it Works	This medication blocks the binding of iodine to the compound that eventually becomes thyroxine (the hormone secreted by the thyroid gland). As a result, decreased effective hormone is produced.
Usual Dosage	30mg daily is the usual adult dose, though this may be lower or higher. A reduced dose is given to children.
Common Side-Effects	Headache, nausea, gastric upsets and skin rashes can occur with carbimazole treatment. Occasionally, blood cell production may be suppressed.
Actions with other Drugs	Nil known.
Pregnancy, Breastfeeding	This medication is not recommended for use in pregnancy. If an anti-thyroid drug has to be used, another medication, Propylthiouracil is preferred. Carbimazole may cause an enlargement of the thyroid gland and lower the thyroid function in the fetus. The drug does pass into breastmilk and if it is used by the mother, the baby should be bottle fed.
Special Features, Comments	Periodic blood tests need to be taken to assess thyroid function and ensure that the blood cell production is normal.

cefaclor

Trade Names	Distaclor
How Available	capsules, syrup
Drug Group	Cephalosporin antibiotic
Prescription	Yes
Major Uses	This antibiotic has a wide variety of uses. Most bacterial respiratory tract infections, urinary tract, skin and ear infections will respond to it.
How it Works	As in similar antibiotics it acts by inhibiting cell wall synthesis in bacteria.
Usual Dosage	250mg three times daily in adults. In children dose depends on age and weight.
Common Side-Effects	Diarrhoea occurs most commonly while nausea and vomiting are less frequent. Skin rashes and more serious allergic problems are rare.
Actions with other Drugs	Cefaclor may interfere with the absorption of the oral contraceptive pill and decrease its efficiency as a contraceptive or cause break-through bleeding. Probenecid will increase the level of cefaclor in the blood.
Pregnancy, Breastfeeding	As a group, cephalosporin antibiotics have been given to large numbers of pregnant women and are generally regarded as safe to use in pregnancy. The drug is excreted in breast milk, but it may be used if the advantages to the mother outweigh possible side-effects.
Special Features, Comments	Nil known. There is no specific interaction with alcohol.

cephalexin

Trade Names	Ceporex, Keflex
How Available	capsule, liquid
Drug Group	Cephalosporin antibiotic
Prescription	Yes
Major Uses	This antibiotic acts on many bacteria and can be used for many infections. Most bacterial respiratory tract infections, urinary tract, skin and ear infections will respond to it. It is sometimes used as a substitute for a penicillin antibiotic, if this is unsuitable.
How it Works	Cephalexin prevents the formation of cell walls in bacteria, as do other members of this group of antibiotics.
Usual Dosage	1-4g per day. As it only lasts a relatively short time in the body it should be given three to four times per day. In children dose depends on weight and age.
Common Side-Effects	Diarrhoea occurs as a result of the activity of the antibiotic on bacteria in the gut. Nausea and vomiting and allergic reactions, rash etc. are much less common.
Actions with other Drugs	This medication reduces the contraceptive efficacy of the oral contraceptive pill. Probenecid will increase cephalexin's level in the blood. Kidney function may be affected if it is used with some other antibiotics.
Pregnancy, Breastfeeding	This drug is widely used in pregnancy and has not been found to have adverse effects. It is thus regarded as being relatively safe. The drug does pass into breast milk, but adverse effects on the baby are unlikely.
Special Features, Comments	Nil of note. Cephalexin has no specific interaction with alcohol.

chloramphenicol

Trade Names	Chloromycetin, Kemicetine, Minims chloramphenicol, Sno Phenicol
How Available	tablet, syrup, ointment, eye drops, ear preparations
Drug Group	Antibiotic
Prescription	Yes
Major Uses	This medication is most commonly used for eye, ear and skin infections, applied to the affected area. It can also be used, and is very effective, for infections in the body such as pneumonia, meningitis and infections of the epiglottis (lower throat). However, occasionally it produces a severe blood disorder called aplastic anaemia if it is given orally or by injection, so it is only used for life-threatening infections.
How it Works	This medication prevents protein from being manufactured within bacteria.
Usual Dosage	The topical preparations are applied three to six times daily, according to instructions.
Common Side-Effects	Occasionally, burning or stinging may occur with drops or ointment. Other allergic problems are not common.
Actions with other Drugs	None are known with the local preparations.
Pregnancy, Breastfeeding	The topical forms of this drug are safe to use during pregnancy and breastfeeding.

chlordiazepoxide

Trade Names	Librium
How Available	tablet
Drug Group	Benzodiazepine
Prescription	Yes
Major Uses	This drug is used to relieve anxiety and tension, relax muscles and to sedate. It can also be used in large doses to treat alcohol withdrawal.
How it Works	Chlordiazepoxide is a benzodiazepine drug. The exact action of these drugs on the central nervous system is not known.
Usual Dosage	10-75mg per day, depending on the type and severity of the problem treated.
Common Side-Effects	The action of this drug in the body can be quite prolonged. As a result, drowsiness during the day can be quite common. There can be difficulty walking and confusion, especially in elderly people. Headache and blurred vision can occur.
Actions with other Drugs	Any drug which has a sedating action will add to the effect of chlordiazepoxide. Sleep drugs, antihistamines, antidepressants, strong analgesics and major tranquillisers will display this additive effect as will alcohol. Cimetidine may lead to a build up of the level of the drug in the blood.
Pregnancy, Breastfeeding	Safety in either pregnancy or breastfeeding has not been shown and the drug should be avoided.
Special Features, Comments	Overdosage is possible with this drug. If a person is excessively drowsy or unresponsive, immediate medical attention should be sought. Long-term use of this drug may have addictive potential. The drug should be ceased slowly, under medical supervision. Alcohol should not be taken with this medication. Driving and hazardous work should be undertaken with extreme caution.

chloroquine

Trade Names	Avloclor, Nivaquine
How Available	tablet, liquid
Drug Group	Anti-malarial
Prescription	Yes

Major Uses
Chloroquine is used for the treatment and prevention of malaria, a parasitic infection transmitted to humans by some types of mosquitoes. It can also be used in rheumatoid arthritis and some other inflammatory conditions.

How it Works
The action of chloroquine in fighting malaria is not known. It is likely to have a number of effects on various stages of the malaria parasite.

Usual Dosage
300mg once per week for prevention of malaria in adults. Lower doses for children. (This should be taken for two weeks before, during and for four weeks after leaving a malaria area.) Treatment of established malaria requires higher doses.

Common Side-Effects
Nausea, headache and abdominal discomfort are the most common side-effects when the tablet is taken in low doses or for short periods of time. If the drug is used in the long-term a number of eye problems can occur. Opacity of the cornea can occur, but resolves if the medication is stopped. Degeneration of the retina is less common, but is not reversible and can cause permanent deterioration in vision.

Actions with other Drugs
Antacids may reduce the absorption of the drug.

Pregnancy, Breastfeeding
This medication is not safe to use during pregnancy or while breastfeeding. Definite abnormalities related to the use of chloroquine have been seen in the fetus.

Special Features, Comments
Intentional or accidental overdosing with chloroquine can be extremely dangerous or even fatal, as in high concentrations the conduction of impulses within the heart is affected. Immediate medical attention is vital if this is suspected. Alcohol may interact with chloroquine and cause liver problems.

chlorothiazide

Trade Names	Saluric
How Available	tablet
Drug Group	Thiazide diuretic (fluid tablet)
Prescription	Yes

Major Uses
This medication is used in the treatment of raised blood pressure. It can also be used in situations in which fluid is retained in the body, such as heart, liver and kidney failure. It will also reduce fluid build up before menstrual periods.

How it Works
Chlorothiazide acts in the kidney to prevent the retention of salts. Thus salts and water pass into the urine, with a net loss of fluid.

Usual Dosage
500mg-1g per day.

Common Side-Effects
Leg cramps are the most common. A range of other side-effects are possible, including dizziness from lowered blood pressure when standing. Due to its effect on the kidney, loss of potassium can be a significant side-effect with long term use. (It is often necessary to use a potassium supplement to prevent a lowered potassium.)

Actions with other Drugs
The potential toxic effects of digitalis are increased if serum potassium is low. Steroid drugs may make potassium loss worse. If used with ACE inhibitors caution should be taken not to cause a too rapid fall in blood pressure. Chlorothiazide may increase lithium levels in the blood, and also decrease the effect of drugs given orally to treat diabetes.

Pregnancy, Breastfeeding
In some situations in pregnancy this drug may be dangerous, and thiazide diuretics are not used. It may cause a reduction of blood flow to the fetus. Milk supply may diminish when it is used by breastfeeding mothers, so it is not commonly used.

Special Features, Comments
Blood tests are often taken at regular intervals to monitor potassium levels. Long-term treatment may cause diabetes, though stopping the drug reverses this. An increase in uric acid level may be caused, and possibly lead to gout. In severe liver disease this medication may be dangerous. The hangover effect of dehydration from alcohol may be made worse by chlorothiazide.

chlorpromazine

Trade Names	Largactil
How Available	tablet, syrup, injection, suppository
Drug Group	Psychiatric drug, anti-nausea drug
Prescription	Yes

Major Uses
Chlorpromazine is a major tranquilliser of the phenothiazine type. It is used to treat mental health problems such as schizophrenia, mania short term confusion or very aggressive behaviour. Chlorpromazine is sometimes used for the treatment of nausea in chronic illness, such as cancer.

How it Works
The phenothiazines have many activities on the brain and the chemicals which transmit messages in the brain (neurotransmitters). Their major action is probably in diminishing the action of one of these, dopamine.

Usual Dosage
This varies considerably with the type and severity of the problem being treated, but the usual dose for longer term treatment is about 25-100mg three times per day. Less of this dose is given for nausea.

Common Side-Effects
Drowsiness, sedation, dizziness, faintness, blurred vision, dry mouth, confusion and movement disorders are the most common side-effects of this drug. The movement problems can be similar to Parkinson's disease with slow movements of the body and a tremor. Involuntary movements of the limbs and tongue may also occur. Weight gain may occur. Other side-effects are possible.

Actions with other Drugs
Any medication which can cause sedation will add to the sedative effects of chlorpromazine. These include sleep drugs, antihistamines, benzodiazepines, antidepressants, strong analgesics, major tranquillisers and alcohol. Chlorpromazine may decrease the beneficial effects of drugs used for Parkinson's disease. Other drugs which have anticholinergic properties may add to the side-effects of chlorpromazine. Seek medical advice before taking any other medication.

Pregnancy, Breastfeeding
After birth, babies of women who have taken chlorpromazine may have movement disorders. Chlorpromazine is generally not used in pregnancy or breastfeeding.

chlorpromazine continued

Special Features,
Comments

If used long term irreversible movement problems may occur. The medication may need to be stopped before surgery. Driving and hazardous work should be performed with great caution. Alcohol should be avoided . Routine blood tests may be necessary to assess liver function.

cholestyramine

Trade Names	Questran
How Available	sachets
Drug Group	Lipid lowering drug
Prescription	Yes
Major Uses	This medication is used as long term treatment to lower blood cholesterol and, sometimes, other blood fats. It can also be used to prevent itching in people with some liver diseases.
How it Works	Bile acids produced by the liver are excreted to help the body absorb fat. They are made up largely of cholesterol. Cholestyramine binds with these bile salts, forming an insoluble complex which is excreted in the faeces, preventing the reabsorption of the bile salts, with a net lowering of serum cholesterol.
Usual Dosage	One to two sachets, two to three times per day.
Common Side-Effects	People taking this medication often complain of its chalky taste. Indigestion, constipation, nausea, abdominal bloating and in some cases offensive-smelling diarrhoea are commonly experienced. Allergic reactions are rare. Fat soluble vitamin absorption may be significantly impaired and supplements may be necessary.
Actions with other Drugs	Cholestyramine interferes with absorption of a wide variety of drugs including anti-coagulants, digitalis, some anti-inflammatory drugs, antibiotics and thyroid drugs. Care must be taken in using these at the same time of day as cholestyramine. It is best to take other medications at different times to cholestyramine.
Pregnancy, Breastfeeding	Safety in the use of this drug in either situation has not been established. Even though side-effects are unlikely, benefits should be weighed against possible problems.
Special Features, Comments	Periodic blood tests are used to check the effectiveness of the medication and to adjust the dose.

cimetidine

Trade Names	Algitec, Dyspament, Galenamet, Peptimax, Phimetin, Tagamet, Ultec, Zita
How Available	tablet
Drug Group	Anti-ulcer drug
Prescription	Yes
Major Uses	Cimetidine is used for the treatment of ulcers in the stomach and duodenum. Following healing of an ulcer, cimetidine is often continued for a longer period to prevent recurrence. It can also be used to decrease the inflammation caused by stomach acid in the oesophagus (reflux oesophagitis).
How it Works	Cimetidine is the first drug in a class called H2 (histamine 2) receptor antagonists. This medication blocks the action of histamine on the cells which produce acid in the stomach. The result is a very large drop in the amount of acid produced. The reduction leads to a decrease in inflammation of the linings of the oesophagus, stomach and duodenum, thus, for example, allowing an ulcer to heal.
Usual Dosage	In the treatment of ulcers the average daily dose is 800mg in adults. This can be given in divided doses or a single dose at night. This dose is usually taken for a month to six weeks, then a lesser dose of 400mg (at night) continued for two to twelve months.
Common Side-Effects	This drug is well tolerated, and the incidence of side-effects is low. Headache, diarrhoea, dizziness, muscle pain and tiredness are possible. Breast enlargement in men can occur.
Actions with other Drugs	Cimetidine may affect the way some other drugs are broken down in the liver, increasing their levels in the blood. These include anti-coagulants, epilepsy drugs, theophylline, beta blockers and some benzodiazepines, including diazepam. Antacids may reduce the absorption of cimetidine.
Pregnancy, Breastfeeding	There has not been any evidence of damage to the fetus or breast-fed babies. If the drug is used, then advantages of using it should outweigh any possible side-effects.
Special Features,	Alcohol and cigarette smoking will impair the healing of ulcers, and thus the effect of cimetidine. Cimetidine should be used with caution in people with impaired kidney function.

ciprofloxacin

Trade Names	Ciproxin
How Available	tablet
Drug Group	Quinolone antibiotic
Prescription	Yes
Major Uses	Ciprofloxacin is an antibiotic which acts on a wide range of bacteria which cause urinary tract infections, gastroenteritis, lung, skin and bone infections. It is very useful for treating gonorrhoea in males and females.
How it Works	The quinolone group of antibiotics inhibit the formation of the genetic building blocks of bacteria (DNA).
Usual Dosage	250-750mg every twelve hours. A single dose of 250mg will effectively treat gonorrhoea. The drug is not recommended for use by children, as it may interfere with growing joint surfaces.
Common Side-Effects	Nausea, vomiting, diarrhoea and rash are the most common, but the drug is well tolerated. Other effects are possible, but rare.
Actions with other Drugs	Ciprofloxacin may increase the level of theophylline in the blood, thus making the side-effects of this drug more common. Antacids may prevent absorption of the drug. Probenecid can increase the level of ciprofloxacin in the blood.
Pregnancy, Breastfeeding	No problems have yet been established in pregnancy, but since it is not recommended for use by children, it is generally not advised in either breastfeeding or pregnancy.

cisapride

Trade Names	Alimix, Prepulsid
How Available	tablet, syrup
Drug Group	Motility agent in the gut
Prescription	Yes
Major Uses	Cisapride is used in the treatment of a number of gastro-enterological motility disorders, the main symptoms of which include early satiety, anorexia, nausea and vomiting.
How it Works	This drug enhances and promotes movement within the gastroenterological tract, by releasing another hormone which promotes motility.
Usual Dosage	5-10mg. three to four times per day is the usual adult dose. In children 0.2mg per kilogram three to four times per day.
Common Side-Effects	Abdominal cramping, abdominal discomfort and diarrhoea may occur as can mild headache and light headedness. Other side-effects are uncommon.
Actions with other Drugs	As the drug increases the rate of emptying of the stomach, many drugs have an increased effect. The effect of sedatives and alcohol may be exaggerated. In contrast, the absorption of digoxin is decreased by cisapride.
Pregnancy, Breastfeeding	Although no adverse effects have been demonstrated in either breastfeeding or pregnancy, the use of cisapride in either is not recommended.
Special Features, Comments	People with kidney or liver insufficiency should take a reduced dose of cisapride as should elderly patients.

clobazam

Trade Names	Frisium
How Available	tablet
Drug Group	Benzodiazepine
Prescription	Yes
Major Uses	Short-term use to relieve anxiety and sleeplessness.
How it Works	The exact action of this drug and of other drugs in the benzodiazepine group is not known. It works on the central nervous system and may add to the effect of some chemicals (neuro-transmitters) as well as possibly having an action of its own.
Usual Dosage	10-30mg per day is the usual adult dose. This medication is not generally prescribed for children.
Common Side-Effects	Sedation, drowsiness and tiredness are the most prominent side-effects and these are common. Dizziness, constipation, difficulty walking and slurred speech are much less frequent.
Actions with other Drugs	Any medication which can cause sedation will add to the sedative side-effects of clobazam. Sleep drugs, antihistamines, antidepressants, strong analgesics, other benzodiazepines and major tranquillisers will display this additive effect as does alcohol.
Pregnancy, Breastfeeding	This drug and some other benzodiazepines may possibly cause developmental defects and clobazam is not recommended, in pregnancy, especially in the first twelve weeks. It can also pass into breast milk and, as children are more susceptible to the adverse effects of these drugs than adults, it is not recommended while breastfeeding.
Special Features, Comments	Long-term use of this drug may have an addiction potential. Excessive sleepiness, or inability to arouse someone with access to this mediation should arouse the suspicion of overdose and medical attention sought. Care should taken in driving or in hazardous work while the drug is being taken. Alcohol will add to clobazam's sedative effect.

clofibrate

Trade Names	Atromid-S
How Available	capsule
Drug Group	Lipid lowering drug
Prescription	Yes
Major Uses	This drug is used mostly to lower the level of cholesterol in the blood, though it can also lower another type of blood fat, triglycerides.
How it Works	The way that this medication works is not fully understood, but it does stop the formation of cholesterol to some extent and also markedly decreases the amount of one type of carrier of blood fats (low density lipoproteins).
Usual Dosage	500mg-1g two to three times per day.
Common Side-Effects	Nausea is the most common. Vomiting, diarrhoea, flatulence and abdominal pain are much rarer. A rash can occur, as can headache, dizziness and tiredness.
Actions with other Drugs	Clofibrate can increase the amount of anti-coagulants in the blood and the effect of this should be checked if the drugs are used together. Similarly, the effect of fluid tablets and diabetic drugs may be increased. Phenytoin may increase the effects of clofibrate.
Pregnancy, Breastfeeding	It is unusual to prescribe this drug in either breastfeeding or pregnancy.
Special Features, Comments	Periodic blood tests are used to check the effectiveness of the medication and to adjust the dose. Gallstones may occur more frequently than normal if this drug is used long-term. Tests on liver function may be necessary.

clomiphene

Trade Names	Clomid, Serophene
How Available	tablet
Drug Group	Fertility drug
Prescription	Yes
Major Uses	This drug is used to artificially induce ovulation in women who wish to become pregnant. It may be used to produce eggs (ova) as part of an IVF (in vitro fertilisation) attempt or for natural fertilisation.
How it Works	Clomiphene stimulates hormone release from the pituitary gland at the base of the brain. The hormones released stimulate the ovaries to produce ova.
Usual Dosage	50mg for five consecutive days in the middle of the menstrual cycle is the usual dose, though this may be increased according to response.
Common Side-Effects	Hot flushes, abdominal discomfort, blurred vision and breast tenderness are the most common, but are usually not severe enough to stop treatment. A rash can occur as well as heavy menstrual periods. Multiple pregnancies (most commonly twins) are more frequent if clomiphene is used.
Actions with other Drugs	No particular interactions have been reported. (The drug is generally used for a short time without other medication.)
Pregnancy, Breastfeeding	The drug should not be used during pregnancy or while breastfeeding. It is important to try and make sure that natural ovulation has not occurred (by taking body temperature) to avoid using the drug in the first weeks of pregnancy.

clomipramine

Trade Names	Anafranil
How Available	tablet
Drug Group	Tricyclic antidepressant
Prescription	Yes
Major Uses	Used for the treatment of depression. The antidepressant effects start after two to three weeks of treatment. Clomipramine can also be used to treat obsessive behaviour and phobias.
How it Works	The exact mode of action of this drug on the central nervous system is not known, though they have widespread effects.
Usual Dosage	The usual starting dose in adults is 50mg. This is usually increased over the period of a few weeks to 50-100mg three times per day. The medication is not usually given to children.
Common Side-Effects	Drowsiness, dry mouth, sweating, dizziness, blurred vision, constipation and difficulty passing urine are common at the start of therapy. Confusion can occur, especially in older people. Other side-effects can occur in individuals.
Actions with other Drugs	All drugs, including alcohol, will add to the sedative effect of clomipramine. These include sleep drugs, antihistamines, other antidepressants, strong analgesics, benzodiazepines and major tranquillisers. Clomipramine and other tricyclic antidepressants should not be used at the same time as another type of antidepressant (MAO inhibitors) because occasionally very serious side-effects may occur. Clomipramine may reduce the effect of some blood pressure reducing drugs. Smoking and barbiturates can reduce the antidepressant effect of this drug.
Pregnancy, Breastfeeding	Safe use of this medication in pregnant women has not been established. Its use should be avoided if possible. Breastfeeding women should also avoid the drug as it can pass into breast milk.
Special Features, Comments	Clomipramine can have serious consequences in overdose situations due to its effects on the heart. Dizziness, blurred vision, dry mouth, agitation, convulsions and lack of arousal may indicate overdosage. Immediate medical attention is imperative. Driving and hazardous work should be undertaken with extreme caution while clomipramine is being taken. Alcohol will increase sedation. It may be necessary to stop this medication prior to surgery.

clonazepam

Trade Names	Rivotril
How Available	tablet, liquid, injection
Drug Group	Benzodiazepine
Prescription	Yes
Major Uses	Unlike most of the other drugs of this group, clonazepam is not used to treat insomnia and anxiety, but is usually used to treat many types of epilepsy (fits) in both children and adults. The intravenous form of the drug can be used in hospitals to treat fits that occur one after another (status epilepticus).
How it Works	The exact action of clonazepam in preventing and treating epilepsy is not known. The drug acts on many nerve junctions and probably exerts its effects this way.
Usual Dosage	In adults and children the starting dose is usually low and increased until the seizures are controlled. For adults 1mg daily is the usual starting dose, in children this is reduced according to age, weight and response to treatment.
Common Side-Effects	When treatment is commenced, sedation is very common, though this side-effect usually decreases substantially as the treatment continues. Tiredness, lack of co-ordination and increased saliva production may occur.
Actions with other Drugs	Any medication which can cause sedation will add to the sedative side-effects of clonazepam. Sleep drugs, antihistamines, antidepressants, strong analgesics and major tranquillisers will display this additive effect as will alcohol. Alcohol should be avoided as it may cause fits. Clonazepam may interfere with the dosages of other antiepileptic drugs, so care should be taken when more than one drug is prescribed.
Pregnancy, Breastfeeding	Clonazepam is used during pregnancy in some cases. Its use may well be beneficial in stopping fits, but its safety for the unborn has not been established. It may be that this medication is the best alternative. If used in breastfeeding, the potential benefits should outweigh potential side-effects.
Special Features, Comments	Side-effects become less prominent the longer the medication is taken. Alcohol should be avoided as this may increase sedation and interfere with the effectiveness of the drug.

clonidine

Trade Names	Catapres, Dixarit
How Available	tablet
Drug Group	Anti-hypertension drug, drug used to prevent migraine
Prescription	Yes
Major Uses	Clonidine is used to lower elevated blood pressure. In low doses the drug can be used to decrease the frequency of migraine headaches. At a similar dose, clonidine is also used to treat flushes which occur during menopause in women.
How it Works	This drug works by diminishing the output of the adrenergic (adrenaline) based nervous system. The net result is a fall in blood pressure. In lower doses it stops some blood vessels from dilating, thus preventing the effects of migraine and menopausal flushing.
Usual Dosage	150-300 micrograms daily (occasionally much higher) for blood pressure. Lower doses for flushing and migraine prevention.
Common Side-Effects	Drowsiness, dry mouth, nausea, vomiting and constipation are the most common, usually when the drug is started. A decrease in blood pressure when standing can also occur, causing dizziness. Other side-effects are rare.
Actions with other Drugs	Clonidine can add to the effect of any drug which causes sedation such as sleep drugs, antihistamines, antidepressants, strong analgesics, major tranquillisers or alcohol. Betablockers may interfere with the blood pressure lowering effect of clonidine.
Pregnancy, Breastfeeding	Increased problems have been demonstrated with clonidine in pregnancy, and it should only be used where benefits clearly outweigh potential side-effects. Its use is not recommended in breastfeeding.
Special Features, Comments	Alcohol should be avoided while taking this drug as its sedative effects may be increased. Clonidine treatment should not be stopped suddenly as this may lead to a dramatic increase in blood pressure.

clotrimazole

Trade Names	Canesten, Lotriderm (with betamethasone), Masnoderm cream
How Available	cream, pessaries
Drug Group	Anti-fungal antibiotic
Prescription	Yes
Major Uses	Clotrimazole is used to treat infections caused by funguses in the skin. These include tinea and ringworm. In addition it can be used to treat fungal infections of the vagina, penis and mouth.
How it Works	Clotrimazole affects the metabolism of the fungus, preventing its normal functioning.
Usual Dosage	Apply to the area 2-3 times per day for skin infections and 1-2 times daily (vaginal infections). Treatment is for 5-10 days.
Common Side-Effects	The only side-effects are rare and include local allergic reactions and burning or stinging. Local allergic reactions are possible.
Actions with other Drugs	None known.
Pregnancy, Breastfeeding	There is no evidence that clotrimazole adversely affects the fetus. The vaginal cream and pessaries are often used to treat fungal infections in pregnant women and are generally considered safe, though this has not been proven. It is safe to use while breastfeeding.
Special Features, Comments	Nil of note.

co-trimoxazole

Trade Names	Bactrim, Chemotrim, Septrin
How Available	tablet, syrup, injection
Drug Group	Antibiotic
Prescription	Yes
Major Uses	This antibiotic is really a combination of two drugs, trimethoprim and sulphamethoxazole. It can be used for a number of bacterial infections in the respiratory system, urinary tract and skin.
How it Works	The two components of this medication inhibit separate components of the metabolism of an essential nutrient (folic acid) in bacteria. By working together, the two drugs not only stop the bacteria from growing, but actually kill it.
Usual Dosage	500mg-1g twice per day. The dose in children varies according to weight and age.
Common Side-Effects	Overall co-trimoxazole is a safe drug and at normal doses the drug is well tolerated. Nausea, vomiting, diarrhoea are the most common side-effects. Allergic side-effects can occur with this medication and may be serious, though this is rare. Other side-effects can occur but are also rare.
Actions with other Drugs	This medication may increase the effect of some oral anti-diabetic drugs, and may lead to low blood glucose (hypoglycaemia). It may increase the effect of anti-coagulants and phenytoin.
Pregnancy, Breastfeeding	The way in which the drug acts may interfere with the developing fetus, so co-trimoxazole is usually avoided in pregnancy. If used a folic acid vitamin supplement is often given as well. The drug passes into the breast milk, so it is usually not used, especially in the first month of breastfeeding.
Special Features, Comments	Recently, there has been concern about the use of this drug combination. In elderly patients, especially those that are ill or taking other medication, severe side-effects, often related to decreased blood cell production (due to suppression of the bone marrow), may occur. A different antibiotic may be more safely prescribed. If co-trimoxazole is used for long periods, folic acid may be given as a vitamin.

codeine

Trade Names	Aspav, Codafen Continus, Kaodene, Migraleve, Panadol Ultra, Paracodol, Propain, Solpadeine, Syndol, Terpoin antitussive, Uniflu
How Available	tablet, liquid
Drug Group	Narcotic analgesic
Prescription	No (Yes for higher strength preparations)
Major Uses	Codeine is an effective analgesic which can be used to treat mild to moderate pain. It can also be effective in treating diarrhoea, and is sometimes used in combination with other medications for this purpose. Persistent dry cough can also be eased with codeine.
How it Works	Codeine acts on specific receptors in the central nervous system and other tissues.
Usual Dosage	20-200mg per day depending on the severity of symptoms.
Common Side-Effects	Side-effects are not common, especially in low doses. Constipation is the most common but nausea and vomiting, dizziness and drowsiness also occur. In higher doses sedation will occur. Other side-effects can occur but are infrequent.
Actions with other Drugs	Any medication which can cause sedation will add to the sedative side-effects of codeine. Sleep drugs, antihistamines, antidepressants, benzodiazepines and major tranquillisers will add to this effect as will alcohol.
Pregnancy, Breastfeeding	Codeine has been used by a large number of pregnant women with no effect to the fetus. It may, however, affect the baby's breathing at birth though oral pain relief is not often used in this situation. The medication can pass through breast milk to the baby and so is to be avoided if possible.
Special Features, Comments	Overdosage with this medication is possible. Drowsiness, difficulty in breathing and excessive sedation suggest overdosage and medical advice should be sought immediately. Codeine can be habit forming if it is taken in large amounts for a prolonged period. Alcohol will increase the sedative effects of codeine. Driving or hazardous work should be undertaken with caution.

colchicine

Trade Names	Not yet available in the UK
How Available	tablet
Drug Group	Drug for gout
Prescription	Yes
Major Uses	Colchicine is used for the treatment of attacks of gout and also to prevent attacks. It is not effective for other types of joint inflammation.
How it Works	Colchicine prevents some of the actions of cells responsible for inflammation in and around joints affected by gout. It does this by interfering with the function within the cell, preventing release of substances causing inflammation.
Usual Dosage	1.0mg is given at the start of treatment for an acute attack of gout. This is followed by 0.5mg every 2-3 hours until the symptoms have subsided or side-effects occur. 0.5mg-1mg daily is the usual dose for the prevention of gout.
Common Side-Effects	Side-effects of colchicine occur very frequently, especially in the doses necessary to stop an attack of gout. These include nausea, vomiting, diarrhoea and abdominal pain. The onset of diarrhoea signals the time to stop the medication. Other side-effects include allergic reactions, rashes and bruising. These are much less common.
Actions with other Drugs	Colchicine may interfere with vitamin B12 absorption, it may also make the effects of sedatives more pronounced.
Pregnancy, Breastfeeding	This drug should not be used in pregnant women, and women should take precautions against falling pregnant while taking the drug, as deformities and birth defects are more common. It passes into the breast milk and is not advised for nursing mothers.
Special Features, Comments	Overdosage of colchicine can be very serious, even fatal. Severe nausea, vomiting, diarrhoea and bleeding from the bowel are signs of overdose. Immediate medical treatment is necessary. Alcohol will increase stomach, especially when higher doses of colchicine are used.

colestipol

Trade Names	Colestid
How Available	sachets
Drug Group	Lipid lowering drug
Prescription	Yes

Major Uses

This medication is used in the long term treatment to lower blood cholesterol and sometimes other blood fats. It can also be used to prevent itching in people with some liver diseases.

How it Works

Bile salts produced by the liver are excreted to help the body absorb fat. They are made up largely of cholesterol. Colestipol binds with these bile salts, forming an insoluble complex which is excreted in the faeces, preventing the reabsorption of the bile salts, resulting in a lowering of blood cholesterol.

Usual Dosage

One to two sachets (10-20g) two or three times per day, depending on blood cholesterol tests. The medication is not usually prescribed for children.

Common Side-Effects

Constipation is the commonest side-effect with colestipol. Other side-effects include abdominal distension and flatulence. People often complain of the chalky taste and bulk of the medication. A rash can occur rarely. Other side-effects are quite rare.

Actions with other Drugs

Colestipol interferes with absorption of a wide variety of drugs (including anti-coagulants, digitalis, some anti-inflammatory drugs, antibiotics and thyroid drugs). Care must be taken in using these at the same time of day as colestipol as the effectiveness of the other medication may be markedly affected. For this reason, they should be taken at other times, not with colestipol.

Pregnancy, Breastfeeding

Safety in the use of this drug in either pregnancy nor breastfeeding has not been established. Even though side-effects are unlikely, benefits should be weighed against possible problems.

Special Features, Comments

Periodic blood tests are used to check the effectiveness of the medication and to adjust the dose.

cyclosporin

Trade Names	Sandimmun
How Available	oral solution
Drug Group	Immune suppression drug
Prescription	Yes
Major Uses	The major use for cyclosporin is to preven the rejection in tissue transplants. It can be used for kidney, heart and other human transplants. It may also be used in situations where other immune system suppressing agents have failed.
How it Works	This drug acts on the function of cells called lymphocytes. These are the cells which are responsible for immune reactions in the body. If these cells are inactivated, then these lymphocytes and the cells they stimulate will not fight the grafted tissue.
Usual Dosage	250-500mg per day in adults. The dose of this drug is given largely on the basis of weight of the patient.
Common Side-Effects	Nausea, vomiting and lack of appetite are common. Also commonly seen are excess growth of facial hair (hirsutism) and impairment of kidney and liver function. Other side-effects are much less frequent.
Actions with other Drugs	Any medication which has been shown to have an adverse effect on the kidney (e.g. some antibiotics) can increase the kidney damaging effect of the drug. A variety of drugs increase the level of cyclosporin in the blood, while others decrease it.
Pregnancy, Breastfeeding	In the past, pregnancy after transplantation would be considered impossible, but this may change in the future. There is a theoretical but unproven risk to the fetus with this drug. The drug is not recommended for breastfeeding mothers.
Special Features, Comments	Often blood levels are checked to ensure that the optimal dose of cyclosporin is being used in each individual.

danazol

Trade Names	Danol
How Available	capsule
Drug Group	Hormone inhibitor
Prescription	Yes

Major Uses
Danazol is mostly used in women with menstrual disorders. Most commonly this is for a condition known as endometriosis, where tissue normally stimulated in the uterus grows in other areas (e.g. around the fallopian tubes). It is also used to treat heavy and excessively painful menstrual periods as well as breast enlargement in males and a rare condition known as hereditary angio-oedema.

How it Works
This medication stops the secretion of hormones from the base of the brain (FSH and LH). These hormones normally stimulate the ovary to produce another hormone, oestrogen. The lack of oestrogen stops the growth of abnormal (and normal) uterine tissue, thus preventing endometriosis.

Usual Dosage
200-800mg. Treatment must commence during menstruation.

Common Side-Effects
Danazol may cause some male hormone side-effects which include weight gain, an increase in facial hair, acne, changes in breast size, hoarseness of the voice and ankle swelling. Nausea is also a feature. Abnormal liver function and thyroid tests may occur and a blood sample is taken to check for these before and during treatment. A rise in blood glucose and blood cholesterol are possible. Menstruation usually ceases during treatment.

Actions with other Drugs
Women who are pregnant or attempting to fall pregnant should not take danazol. There is a definite danger of deformity to the fetus, especially females. The drug is not recommended for breastfeeding women. Oral contraceptives should not be used concurrently with danazol. The effect of anti-coagulants may be increased with danazol treatment.

Pregnancy, Breastfeeding
Blood tests may be taken if the medication is to be used for long periods (months).

dexamethasone

Trade Names	Decadron, Maxidex, Maxitrol, Otomize, Sofradex
How Available	tablet, injection, ear and eye drops (combination), nasal spray (combination)
Drug Group	Corticosteroid
Prescription	Yes

Major Uses

Dexamethasone is used for a number of inflammatory conditions in the eyes and ears. The injectable form may be used to decrease inflammation when injected into joints. After head injury and neurosurgery, injected dexamethasone is a help to prevent brain swelling. It can be used for severe asthma. Tablets can be taken orally if the body is deficient in corticosteroids, which are vital for proper functioning. Dexamethasone is sometimes used if extra corticosteroids are necessary. Dexamethasone has many other uses in some inflammatory and blood disorders.

How it Works

Dexamethasone is very similar to a hormone produced by the body and it replaces this natural substance when taken by mouth. The exact way that it reduces inflammation in the skin and other sites is unknown, though one important effect is preventing cells which cause inflammation from arriving at the inflamed tissue.

Usual Dosage

This varies widely according to the nature and severity of the condition being treated. Topical preparations are used two to three times per day.

Common Side-Effects

All corticosteroids can produce a similar range of side-effects. If taken orally these include indigestion, nausea, weight gain, acne, weakness and thin bones. Peptic ulcer may occur. These side-effects usually occur with long-term treatment. Mood changes are possible with higher doses. Topical preparations can lead to thinning of the skin if used continuously. A rash may also occur. Use of topical medications does not lead to similar side-effects as little is absorbed.

Actions with other Drugs

Barbiturates, phenytoin, the oral contraceptive pill and rifampicin may decrease the effect of dexamethasone. Dexamethasone may

continued over page...

impair the control of diabetes with insulin or oral tablets and also interfere with blood pressure control. Vaccination should be delayed till dexamethasone treatment is completed, if possible.

Pregnancy, Breastfeeding

Corticosteroids, given orally, may lead to birth defects, and decrease the baby's weight. At the end of pregnancy, if the baby is about to be born prematurely, a short course of corticosteroids may be given to the mother to help prevent respiratory distress in the baby. Otherwise, dexamethasone is used only if absolutely necessary. It is generally avoided in breastfeeding also, as it does pass into breastmilk.

Special Features, Comments

Blood tests at regular intervals may be necessary. Checks should be made from time to time to ensure that glaucoma (raised eye pressure) and diabetes are not present. Alcohol may increase the chance of peptic ulcer if taken with oral dexamethasone.

dexfenfluramine

Trade Names	Adifax
How Available	capsule
Drug Group	Drug for weight loss
Prescription	Yes
Major Uses	Dexfenfluramine is used for weight loss as an adjunct to diet.
How it Works	This drug increases the level of a substance known as serotonin, around the part of the brain which is responsible for appetite control. This inhibits appetite, making a reduction in food intake easier and eventually leading to a reduction in weight.
Usual Dosage	15mg twice per day.
Common Side-Effects	Drowsiness, tiredness, dry mouth and mild depression are the most commonly encountered side-effects. These are usually minimal and people generally get used to them quickly.
Actions with other Drugs	Dexfenfluramine should not be given with other appetite suppressing drugs. It may also increase the effect of some blood pressure reducing drugs, drugs used to treat diabetes and some sedatives.
Pregnancy, Breastfeeding	This medication is not recommended for use in pregnant women or women who are breastfeeding.
Special Features, Comments	Treatment is usually only for three continuous months. Treatment will only be effective if accompanied by a decrease in dietary intake. Long-term weight reduction will only occur if patterns of food use change.

dextropropoxyphene

Trade Names	Cosalgesic, Distalgesic, Doloxene
How Available	tablet
Drug Group	Narcotic analgesic
Prescription	Yes
Major Uses	Dextropropoxyphene is used in combination with paracetamol for the relief of mild to moderate pain. The paracetamol component can be used to reduce fever.
How it Works	Dextropropoxyphene is a mild narcotic analgesic. It acts on specific receptors in the central nervous system responsible for the perception of pain.
Usual Dosage	2 tablets, three to four times per day.
Common Side-Effects	Most frequently seen are dizziness, sedation, constipation and nausea and vomiting. Other side-effects are not common.
Actions with other Drugs	Any medication which can cause sedation will add to the sedative side-effects of dextropropoxyphene. Sleep drugs, antihistamines, antidepressants, strong analgesics, major tranquillisers and benzodiazepines will display this additive effect as will alcohol. This medication may also increase the effects of anti-coagulants.
Pregnancy, Breastfeeding	The drug is suspected of harmful effects in the fetus and is not recommended for use in pregnancy nor in breastfeeding women.
Special Features, Comments	Overdosage can be a problem with this drug. Drowsiness and inability to arouse someone should raise the suspicion of overdosage. In overdose situations a large dose of paracetamol will also have been consumed. This can have very harmful effects on the liver and kidneys. Immediate medical advice should be sought. Dextropropoxyphene can be habit forming if used for prolonged periods of time. Alcohol will increase the sedative effects of dextroproxyphene. Driving and hazardous work should be undertaken with caution.

diazepam

Trade Names	Diazemuls, Valium
How Available	tablet, injection
Drug Group	Benzodiazepine
Prescription	Yes
Major Uses	Diazepam is used for short-term control of anxiety, relief of muscle spasm, sedation and to induce sleep. It can also be used to control fits and prolonged muscle spasm of tetanus as well as preventing some of the severe effects of drug withdrawal.
How it Works	The exact action of this group of drugs is unknown but it is thought to depress the activity in that part of the brain which controls emotion.
Usual Dosage	Usual dosage is 5-10mg per day but up to 40mg may be used for treating some problems.
Common Side-Effects	Day-time drowsiness, dizziness, unsteadiness and weakness are the most common. Confusion and sometimes paradoxical rage and anxiety can occur, but are infrequent. Elderly people are more likely to experience side-effects.
Actions with other Drugs	Any medication which can cause sedation will add to the sedative side-effects of diazepam. Sleep drugs, antihistamines, antidepressants, other benzodiazepines, strong analgesics and major tranquillisers will display this additive effect as will alcohol. Cimetidine can interfere with the breakdown of diazepam. Diazepam leads to an increased effect of digoxin as well as phenytoin.
Pregnancy, Breastfeeding	Though it has been used in pregnancy, this medication should be avoided unless absolutely necessary. The drug passes into breast milk and its use is not advised in breastfeeding mothers.
Special Features, Comments	Regular, continual use can decrease the effectiveness of diazepam and benzodiazepines. Overdosage with this medication is possible. Excessive tiredness or profound sleepiness should raise the possibility of overdosage. Immediate medical attention is advisable. Prolonged use has the potential to cause dependency. Alcohol may add to the sedative effects of the drug. Diazepam can cause reduced alertness, so driving and dangerous work should be undertaken with care.

diclofenac

Trade Names	Arthrotec, Diclomax Retard, Diclozip, Flamrase, Motifene, Rhumalgen, Valenac, Volraman, Voltarol Ophtha, Voltarol
How Available	tablet, gel, suppositories, injections
Drug Group	NSAID (non-steroidal anti-inflammatory drug)
Prescription	Yes

Major Uses

Diclofenac is a commonly used NSAID which is used to reduce pain, inflammation and joint discomfort in a variety of situations. These include soft tissue and joint inflammation, and pain associated with menstrual periods.

How it Works

This drug prevents the action of substances (prostaglandins) which act on local tissues to produce pain and inflammation.

Usual Dosage

25-50mg two to three times per day. The gel should be applied two to three times per day. It is not recommended for use in children.

Common Side-Effects

All NSAIDs produce gastro-intestinal symptoms to some degree. These most commonly are nausea, vomiting and upper abdominal pain. Diarrhoea is less frequent. It is rare, but possible for diclofenac to produce an ulcer in the stomach or duodenum and this may bleed. (For this reason any person with a history of ulcer disease should avoid diclofenac and NSAIDs generally.) Headache and dizziness may occur as may other side-effects, but they are rare. Local skin irritation can be caused by the gel.

Actions with other Drugs

Use of this drug with aspirin or steroids may increase the chances of peptic ulcer and bleeding. Aspirin may also reduce the level of diclofenac in the blood. Digoxin may increase the level of diclofenac in the blood. It may interfere with the action of anti-coagulant drugs.

Pregnancy, Breastfeeding

Diclofenac theoretically may cause some problems in fetal development and may also interfere with the baby's blood circulation in the heart late in pregnancy. Thus it is not recommended. It has not been shown to cross over to the infant in breast milk, but its use in breastfeeding should be discussed with your doctor.

Special Features, Comments

Alcohol will increase the irritation of the stomach caused by diclofenac. Diclofenac is not to be used in people with a history of peptic ulcers. This medication should be given with caution in people with impaired liver function or in people with heart failure. Diclofenac may interfere with bleeding and this should be considered before surgery or dental work.

dicyclomine

Trade Names	Diarrest, Infacol-C colic syrup, Kolanticon, Merbentyl
How Available	tablet, liquid
Drug Group	Bowel anti-spasm drug
Prescription	Yes
Major Uses	This drug is used alone (Merbentyl) and in combination for the treatment of pain and discomfort related to spasm of smooth muscle in the walls of the bowel (colic, or colicky abdominal pain). It is often used to treat infantile colic.
How it Works	Dicyclomine acts directly on the muscle of the wall of the bowel to produce its action. It also works on part of the nervous system to help with wind, indigestion and diarrhoea.
Usual Dosage	30-150mg per day. Usually 4 doses per day.
Common Side-Effects	Side-effects most commonly reported are those due to the nervous system (anti-cholinergic) effects of the drug. These are dry mouth, blurred vision, constipation, drowsiness and sometimes difficulty in passing urine. Other effects are rare. In very young infants (less than three months), breathing problems have occurred occasionally if the syrup has been used.
Actions with other Drugs	Any medication which can cause sedation will add to the sedative side-effects of dicyclomine. Sleep drugs, antihistamines, anti-depressants, strong analgesics and major tranquillisers will display this additive effect as does alcohol.
Pregnancy, Breastfeeding	No definite problems have been shown to occur with dicyclomine in pregnancy or breastfeeding, but its use should be of clear value before it is prescribed.
Special Features, Comments	Alcohol will increase the sedative effects of the drug. Driving and dangerous tasks should be performed with caution.

diethylpropion

Trade Names	Tenuate Dospan
How Available	tablet
Drug Group	Drug for weight loss
Prescription	Yes
Major Uses	Diethylpropion is used as an adjunct to diet to achieve weight loss.
How it Works	This medication acts on the central nervous system to decrease food intake.
Usual Dosage	75mg per day.
Common Side-Effects	The drug has stimulating effects on the body, and can cause jitteriness, nervousness and lack of sleep. Palpitations and a rise in blood pressure can occur, and it should be used cautiously in people with heart problems or raised blood pressure. Nausea and vomiting are potential problems. A wide variety of less common side-effects have occurred.
Actions with other Drugs	This medication can act with some anti-depressants. It can make the stimulant effects of coffee and nicotine more pronounced. It should not be given with other weight control tablets. Diethylpropion may counter-act the effect of blood pressure lowering agents.
Pregnancy, Breastfeeding	This medication is not usually recommended for use in pregnancy or breastfeeding.
Special Features, Comments	Treatment is usually only for three continuous months. Treatment will only be effective if accompanied by a decrease in dietary intake. Long-term weight reduction will only occur if patterns of food use change. It should not be used in people with raised eye pressure (glaucoma) or in people with a history of agitation or drug abuse. Driving and hazardous work should be undertaken with caution.

CHOPRA & ASSOCIATES
DENTAL SURGERY

YOUR DENTAL CHECK UP IS NOW DUE

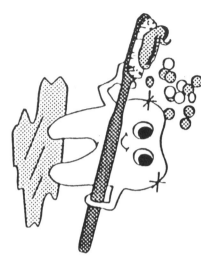

To book an appointment please

TELEPHONE

your practice on:-

SITTINGBOURNE
'Sutton House' No 5 London Road
on (01795) 477224

~ ~ ~ ~ ~ ~ ~ ~ ~ ~

SWANSCOMBE
'Hews House' No 23 High Street
on (01322) 386688

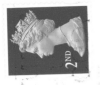

POST

Mrs I Lorkins

12 Gadby Road
Sittingbourne
Kent

ME10 1TF

digoxin

Trade Names	Lanoxin
How Available	tablet, syrup
Drug Group	Heart drug
Prescription	Yes

Major Uses
This medication has been used for centuries. It is of use in most cases of heart failure and can also be used for some specific type of fast heart rhythms to control the heart rate.

How it Works
Digoxin actually assists the heart muscle to act more effectively and so to pump blood around the body. It also slows conduction of the electrical impulse which causes each heart beat, thus lowering the number of heart beats per minute.

Usual Dosage
0.125 to 0.25mg per day in adults, by single dose. In children the dose is administered according to age and weight.

Common Side-Effects
Nausea, tiredness, disturbances of vision and confusion are relatively common. Missed heart beats are also possible. The dose that leads to the beneficial effects of digoxin is close to the toxic dose of the drug. Any side-effects or suspected side-effects should be brought to the attention of a doctor as soon as possible.

Actions with other Drugs
Low potassium levels in the blood can make the toxic effects of digoxin more likely. This can occur due to the use of fluid tablets (diuretics) and is the most common drug interaction with digoxin. (Diuretics and digoxin are often used together for heart failure.) It is important to monitor potassium levels in the blood and give potassium supplements if necessary or as a precaution. Digoxin affects blood levels of a number of medications such as heart rhythm agents, calcium channel blockers, lithium and quinidine.

Pregnancy, Breastfeeding
Many pregnant women and breastfeeding women have taken digoxin, and no ill effects have been demonstrated. They are generally considered safe for use in pregnancy and breastfeeding.

Special Features, Comments
The level of digoxin in the blood may need checking from time to time (as does the level of potassium in the blood). Overdosage with digoxin can occur relatively easily and can be very serious, even fatal. Weakness, palpitations and chest pain are possible symptoms. Immediate medical help is vital.

diltiazem

Trade Names	Adizem, Britiazim, Dilzem, Metazem, Tildiem
How Available	tablet, slow release tablet
Drug Group	Calcium channel blocker
Prescription	Yes
Major Uses	Diltiazem is used to lower blood pressure and also to prevent angina pectoris (inadequate supply of blood to the heart). It is not effective in treating an attack of angina once it has started, as it does not act rapidly enough taken orally.
How it Works	Calcium channel blockers are thought to prevent the flow of calcium in the walls of smooth muscle cells which line small arteries. This decreases blood pressure, increases flow through the arteries and prevents spasm of the walls of arteries (which occurs in the heart in some attacks of angina).
Usual Dosage	120-360mg per day in three doses. Diltiazem is not generally used in children. Slow release tablets are generally used twice per day.
Common Side-Effects	Headache, ankle swelling, rash and nausea are the most frequent, though many rarer side-effects are possible. They usually occur at the start of treatment and disappear or decrease with time.
Actions with other Drugs	Diltiazem increases the effects of drugs which lower blood pressure. Beta-blocker medications can act at a similar place in the heart conduction system to lead to a serious slowing of heart rate. Heart conduction problems can also occur if diltiazem is used with digoxin or amiodarone. Cimetidine increases the effects of diltiazem.
Pregnancy, Breastfeeding	Diltiazem theoretically can cause fetal abnormalities and freely crosses into breast milk, so it is not recommended in either pregnancy or breastfeeding.
Special Features, Comments	Alcohol may accentuate the blood pressure lowering effects of diltiazem. Diltiazem should be used cautiously in people with poor cardiac function e.g. severe heart failure. It may make this problem worse.

diphenoxylate with atropine

Trade Names	Lomotil
How Available	tablet, liquid
Drug Group	Anti-diarrhoeal drug
Prescription	Yes
Major Uses	Diphenoxylate is used for the symptomatic treatment of diarrhoea.
How it Works	This medication reduces contraction in the large bowel. As a result, there is increased reabsorption of fluid in the large bowel with a reduction in number of stools.
Usual Dosage	Two tablets 3 to 4 times daily.
Common Side-Effects	Drowsiness, confusion, headache and dizziness can occur. The cessation of colon activity can have a rare but serious side-effect (toxic megacolon). The side-effects of this medication can be more pronounced in children, so it is not recommended for children less than twelve years of age.
Actions with other Drugs	Any medication which can cause sedation will add to the sedative side-effects of diphenoxylate. Sleep drugs, antihistamines, anti-depressants, strong analgesics, benzodiazepines and major tranquillisers will display this additive effect as does alcohol. One type of drug used for depression (mono-amine oxidase inhibitor) can cause a dramatic rise in blood pressure if used with diphenoxylate.
Pregnancy, Breastfeeding	This drug should not be given during pregnancy near the time of delivery as it may cause respiratory problems for the infant. It is not recommended for breastfeeding mothers.
Special Features, Comments	Alcohol may cause an increase in sedation. Overdosage with this medication is possible. A dry mouth and excessive sleeplessness should raise the possibility of overdose. If suspected, immediate attention should be sought. Driving and dangerous work should be undertaken with caution.

disopyramide

Trade Names	Dirythmin SA, Rhythmodan
How Available	tablet, injection
Drug Group	Heart rhythm drug
Prescription	Yes
Major Uses	Disopyramide is most commonly used after heart attacks which are complicated by heart rhythm disturbances. It can also be used for a variety of other heart rhythm problems.
How it Works	This medication exerts a number of actions on the transmission of the electrical impulse through the heart. The net result of these effects is to prolong the amount of time before certain areas of the heart can be stimulated by a further electrical impulse.
Usual Dosage	300-800mg per day in divided doses is the usual adult daily dose. The medication is not usually prescribed in children, though a reduced dose will be necessary if it is used, depending on weight and age.
Common Side-Effects	Dry mouth, blurred vision and constipation are the most common side-effects with disopyramide. A rash, nausea, dizziness and tiredness are less frequent. Rare, but potentially serious side-effects (especially if they occur after a heart attack) are a dramatic fall in blood pressure and heart failure.
Actions with other Drugs	Other medications which lower blood pressure can increase these potential side-effects of disopyramide. Phenytoin may reduce the effect of disopyramide. Use of other rhythm controlling drugs with disopyramide requires considerable caution.
Pregnancy, Breastfeeding	Although no specific problems have been demonstrated with disopyramide in pregnancy or breastfeeding, the medication is generally not used unless absolutely necessary.
Special Features, Comments	Disopyramide should not be used in people with heart failure or very low blood pressure. The drug can make some rhythm disturbances worse. A fall in blood glucose can occur. People with liver and kidney disease may require a lower dose.

dithranol

Trade Names	Dithrocream, Dithrolan, Psoradrate, Psorin
How Available	ointment, cream
Drug Group	Drug for psoriasis
Prescription	Yes
Major Uses	This medication is used for the treatment of severe psoriasis (a skin condition of unknown cause, but characterised by an increased turnover of cells in the skin).
How it Works	Dithranol inhibits the actions of some enzymes in skin cells and decreases the turnover rate of skin cells.
Usual Dosage	The strength of the cream and the duration of application vary according to the severity of the disease. A thin film is applied for up to thirty minutes per day and then washed off. An improvement can occur in a few days, but the full benefit is not visible for some weeks.
Common Side-Effects	Skin irritation is very common and may require lowering the dose or stopping the medication. A rash may occur.
Actions with other Drugs	Medications which increase the skin's sensitivity to light may interact with dithranol. These include coal tar, some antibiotics (e.g. tetracyclines), diuretics and phenothiazines.
Pregnancy, Breastfeeding	There is no proof of safety in pregnancy or breastfeeding, so use is not advised unless absolutely necessary.
Special Features, Comments	The medication should be applied with gloves and areas of blistered skin should not be treated. The medication may stain clothes and bed-linen.

domperidone

Trade Names	Motilium
How Available	tablet
Drug Group	Anti-nausea drug
Prescription	Yes
Major Uses	This medication is used for the treatment of nausea and vomiting caused by gastro-intestinal causes. Domperidone is also used to treat nausea in chronic illness e.g. cancer. It is not effective for motion sickness or other causes of nausea.
How it Works	Domperidone acts directly on the gastro-intestinal tract to exert its effects. It also may act on the base of the brain to decrease the action of a naturally occurring substance (dopamine).
Usual Dosage	10mg three to four times daily.
Common Side-Effects	As this medication does not actually cross into the brain (as do other anti-nausea drugs) it has few common side-effects in prescribed doses. Specifically, it does not usually cause drowsiness. Occasional cramps and dry mouth are rare. The medication can possibly interfere with a mother's milk supply.
Actions with other Drugs	Some anti-cholinergic drugs may decrease the effectiveness of domperidone as may some narcotic analgesics.
Pregnancy, Breastfeeding	Domperidone is not recommended for use either in pregnancy or breastfeeding, though no specific problems have been found.

dothiepin

Trade Names	Prothiaden
How Available	tablet, capsule
Drug Group	Tricyclic antidepressant
Prescription	Yes
Major Uses	This medication is used for the treatment of depression. It also encourages sleep and reduces anxiety. The antidepressant effects start after two to three weeks of treatment.
How it Works	The exact mode of action of this group of drugs on the central nervous system is not known.
Usual Dosage	75-150mg, usually in one dose at night.
Common Side-Effects	Drowsiness, dry mouth, sweating, blurred vision, constipation and difficulty passing urine are common when Prothiaden is started or the dose increased. Other side-effects have been reported in individual people taking this medication.
Actions with other Drugs	All drugs, including alcohol which have a sedative effect will have an additive effect on dothiepin. Sleep drugs, antihistamines, other antidepressants, strong analgesics, benzodiazepines and major tranquillisers are the most common examples. Dothiepin and other tricyclic anti-depressants should not be used at the same time as another type of anti-depressant (MAO inhibitors) as occasionally very serious side-effects may occur. Dothiepin may reduce the effect of some blood pressure reducing drugs. Smoking may interfere with therapy.
Pregnancy, Breastfeeding	Safe use of this medication in pregnant women has not been established. Its use should be avoided if possible. Nursing mothers should also avoid the drug as it can pass into breast milk.
Special Features, Comments	All tricyclic antidepressants including dothiepin can have serious consequences if an overdose is taken as eventually they will have a profound effect on the heart. Dizziness, blurred vision, dry mouth, agitation, convulsions and lack of arousal should give rise to suspicion of overdosage. Immediate medical attention is imperative. Due to its sedative properties it is important not to drive or do hazardous work until the effect of the drug is established. Alcohol will increase sedation.

doxepin

Trade Names	Sinequan
How Available	tablet, capsule
Drug Group	Tricyclic antidepressant
Prescription	Yes

Major Uses
This medication is used for the treatment of depression. It also encourages sleep and reduces agitation, which can be beneficial. The antidepressant effects start after 2-3 weeks of treatment.

How it Works
The exact mode of action of this group of drugs on the central nervous system is not known.

Usual Dosage
Initially 10-25mg increasing to 75-150mg at night. Elderly at lower doses.

Common Side-Effects
When doxepin is started or the dose increased the following side-effects are common. They include drowsiness, dry mouth, sweating, dizziness, blurred vision, constipation and difficulty passing urine. Other side-effects can occur in individual people.

Actions with other Drugs
All drugs, including alcohol which have a sedative effect will have an additive effect on doxepin. Sleep drugs, antihistamines, other antidepressants, strong analgesics, benzodiazepines and major tranquillisers are the most common examples. Doxepin and other tricyclic antidepressants should not be used at the same time as another type of antidepressant (MAO inhibitors) as occasionally very serious side-effects may occur. Doxepin may reduce the effect of some blood pressure reducing drugs. Smoking and barbiturates can reduce the antidepressant effect of this drug.

Pregnancy, Breastfeeding
Safe use of this medication in pregnant women has not been established. Its use should be avoided if possible. Breastfeeding women should also avoid the drug as it can pass into breast milk.

Special Features, Comments
All tricyclic antidepressants including doxepin can have serious consequences if an overdose is taken as eventually they will have a profound effect on the heart. Dizziness, blurred vision, dry mouth, agitation, convulsions and lack of arousal should give rise to suspicion of overdosage. Immediate medical attention is imperative. Due to its sedative properties it is important not to drive or do dangerous work until the effect of the doxepin is established. Alcohol will increase sedation.

doxycycline

Trade Names	Nordox, Vibramycin
How Available	tablet
Drug Group	Tetracycline antibiotic
Prescription	Yes
Major Uses	Doxycycline is an antibiotic effective against a wide variety of bacteria. It is used for ear, throat and respiratory tract infections. It can be used for some sexually transmitted diseases (Chlamydia) and is effective in prostate gland infections. Its antibacterial activity is used to treat acne.
How it Works	This drug acts by preventing the formation of protein within bacteria. It prevents bacteria from growing, rather than killing the bacteria.
Usual Dosage	50-200mg per day is the usual adult dose depending on the type and severity of the problem being treated. The drug is not usually given to children less than eight years.
Common Side-Effects	Nausea is probably the most common side-effect and for this reason it is recommended that the medication is given with food. Diarrhoea and a rash on exposure to the sun are also possible. Many other side-effects can occur, but are less likely. Also, the tablet may get caught in the oesophagus.
Actions with other Drugs	Antacids can decrease the absorption of doxycycline. Some epilepsy drugs can decrease its effect. Doxycycline can interfere with the oral contraceptive pill, and anti-coagulant drugs. Tetracyclines may also interfere with the action of penicillin and are not usually given at the same time.
Pregnancy, Breastfeeding	This group of drugs can interfere with the growth and development of teeth in the fetus, and in children less than age eight years. Discolouration of teeth can occur if children are given doxycycline. It may cause retarded growth of bones as well. It is not recommended for use by pregnant or breastfeeding women.
Special Features, Comments	Nil of note. There is no interaction with alcohol, except that both can cause irritation to the stomach.

econazole

Trade Names	Econacort, Ecostatin, Gyno-Pevaryl, Pevaryl
How Available	syrup, pessary, powder, cream, lotion
Drug Group	Anti-fungal antibiotic
Prescription	Yes
Major Uses	Econazole is an anti-fungal antibiotic with a wide variety of uses against many types of funguses, including tinea, ringworm and athlete's foot. Pessaries are used for vaginal infections and syrups for mouth infections.
How it Works	Econazole affects the metabolism of the cell membrane of funguses, preventing their normal functioning.
Usual Dosage	Apply to the affected area up to three times daily. Treatment should continue for several days following cessation of symptoms to prevent recurrence.
Common Side-Effects	These are uncommon. Occasionally, a local stinging may occur, or redness and itchiness to the skin. Local allergic reactions are possible.
Actions with other Drugs	None known.
Pregnancy, Breastfeeding	There is no evidence that this drug adversely affects the fetus. The vaginal cream and pessaries are often used to treat fungal infections in pregnant women and are generally considered safe, though this has not been proven. It is safe to use while breastfeeding.

enalapril

Trade Names	Innovace, Innozide
How Available	tablet
Drug Group	ACE inhibitor (angiotensin converting enzyme inhibitor)
Prescription	Yes

Major Uses Enalapril is most commonly used for the long-term treatment of raised blood pressure. In addition it is used to reduce the workload of the heart and can be effective in heart failure.

How it Works Enalapril works mainly by preventing the action of the enzyme angiotensin converting enzyme in transforming angiotensin I to angiotensin II. Angiotensin II is a very active substance which leads to a marked increase in blood pressure, so stopping its formation generally leads to a reduction in blood pressure. Reduced blood pressure can diminish the workload of the heart and improve its function.

Usual Dosage Enalapril is usually given in a low dose 2.5-5mg at first and then increased according to the response of the patient. Up to 40mg per day can be used. This medication has not been proven safe for children and is not recommended for their use.

Common Side-Effects Headache, dizziness, tiredness are the most common side-effects with enalapril. A rash and persistent dry cough can occur, and may require ceasing treatment. Other side-effects are much less common.

Actions with other Drugs Excessive lowering of blood pressure may occur in people taking other blood pressure lowering tablets or fluid tablets. Enalapril increases the level of lithium in the blood. Some anti-inflammatory drugs may interfere with the effectiveness of enalapril.

Pregnancy, Breastfeeding Enalapril may cause birth defects and is not generally used in pregnant women. It is also not considered safe for use during breastfeeding, though no specific problems have been demonstrated.

Special Features, Comments Enalapril may worsen kidney function in people suffering from kidney disease. It may raise the level of potassium in the blood especially in people taking fluid tablets that spare potassium. From time to time, checks on blood chemistry should be made. Alcohol may make some side-effects worse.

ergotamine

Trade Names	Cafergot, Lingraine, Medihaler-ergotamine, Migril
How Available	tablet, suppository, inhaler, injection
Drug Group	Anti-migraine drug
Prescription	Yes
Major Uses	Ergotamine is used at the beginning of a migraine headache to prevent the headache from progressing. It is of limited effectiveness if the headache is established.
How it Works	This medication works by constricting veins on the outside of the brain. Nerve endings on these veins are responsible for the migraine headache.
Usual Dosage	1-2mg at the onset of headache or when a warning that a headache is imminent is the usual adult dose. This is repeated every 30 minutes till the headache subsides. No more than 6mg per 24 hours or 10mg per week is recommended. This medication is not generally used in children.
Common Side-Effects	Nausea, vomiting ,unusual sensations and coolness in the arms and legs, muscle pain and stiffness may occur. Chest pain can occur infrequently. Other side-effects are rare.
Actions with other Drugs	Drugs which decrease circulation to the body (e.g. betablockers) may increase the blood vessel constricting side-effects of ergotamine. Use of erythromycin at the same time as ergotamine may also do this. The contents of some combination preparations used for colds etc. may cause serious increases in blood pressure.
Pregnancy, Breastfeeding	It is generally not safe to take ergotamine during pregnancy as it may cause uterine contractions and premature labour. (A type of ergotamine has been used to stop bleeding after childbirth.) Ergotamine is not generally recommended for nursing mothers.
Special Features, Comments	Alcohol may cause migraine, so it is best avoided. Regular use of ergotamine can lead to circulation problems in the hands and feet, especially if the recommended upper limits of dosage are exceeded. Ergotamine should not be used in people with impaired circulation to the heart or limbs, liver and kidney disease or severely raised blood pressure. An overdose of this medication requires prompt medical attention in hospital.

erythromycin

Trade Names	Arpimycin, Benzamycin, Erycen, Erymax, Erythrocin, Erythroped, Ilosone, Rommix, Stiemycin, Zineryt
How Available	tablet, liquid, injection
Drug Group	Antibiotic
Prescription	Yes
Major Uses	This antibiotic is used for a wide variety of bacterial infections caused by a number of organisms. It is used in respiratory, ear, skin and tissue infections, as well as some types of pneumonia. It can be also be used for some sexually transmitted diseases and to treat whooping cough.
How it Works	Erythromycin works by preventing the manufacture of protein within bacteria. At low concentrations it stops the bacteria from growing, at higher concentrations it kills the bacteria.
Usual Dosage	1-4g per day in divided doses is the usual adult dose depending on the nature and severity of the infection. In children age and weight are important in determining dose.
Common Side-Effects	Nausea, vomiting, loss of appetite and abdominal pain are common. A rash can occur as can other allergic reactions. Occasionally some types of erythromycin can interfere with liver function. Other side-effects are rare.
Actions with other Drugs	Erythromycin can increase the blood levels (and thus side-effects) of carbamazepine, anti-coagulants, theophylline, and digoxin. Erythromycin may increase the drug levels of some anti-histamines and rarely the combination may cause heart rhythm problems.
Pregnancy, Breastfeeding	This medication has been used extensively in pregnant women and there is no evidence of adverse effects on the fetus. Accordingly, it is generally considered safe, but used only if necessary. At normal doses, it is not thought that erythromycin will affect a breastfed baby.
Special Features, Comments	Erythromycin should be avoided in people who are known to have liver disease.

ethinyloestradiol

Trade Names	BiNovum, Brevinor, Cilest, Eugynon, Femodene ED, Loestrin 20, Logynon, Logynon ED, Marvelon, Mercilon, Minulet, Neocon, Norimin, Ortho-Novin 1/50, Ovran, Ovranette, Ovysmen, Schering PC4, Synphase, Tri-Minulet, Triadene, Trinordiol, Trimarin
How Available	tablet
Drug Group	Oral contraceptive (female sex hormone)
Prescription	Yes
Major Uses	Ethinyloestradiol is most commonly used as one of two components to many oral contraceptive pills. It is combined with a variety of progestagen hormones. (Ethinyloestradiol is an oestrogen.) It can also be used for hormone replacement at and after menopause, to control irregular or excessive menstrual bleeding and in a variety of other medical problems.
How it Works	The contraceptive effect of this medication is due to its ability to prevent hormones (secreted from the pituitary gland at the base of the brain) from being released. As a result, the ovary is not stimulated and no ova are released. Oestrogens stimulate a wide variety of other cells in the female body, most importantly the lining of the uterus (the endometrium) and this stimulation is responsible for the other therapeutic effects of the drug.
Usual Dosage	10-20 micrograms per day for hormone replacement is the average dose for most women. A higher dose 30-50 micrograms is the range of dose used in combined oral contraceptive pills.
Common Side-Effects	Nausea and vomiting are the most common side-effects of this drug. Breast tenderness and a gain in weight are common problems with combined oral contraceptives. Abdominal cramps, change to skin colour, a reduction (or occasional increase) in menstrual bleeding, bleeding in between cycles, increased frequency of migraine headaches, change in mood, decreased milk supply in breastfeeding women, altered liver function and a rise in blood pressure may occur.
Actions with other Drugs	Some antibiotics can reduce the absorbed amount of oestrogen and decrease the contraceptive effect or cause breakthrough bleeding. The effect of blood pressure and blood glucose lowering drugs may be offset by ethinyloestradiol. Smoking increases the risk of some serious side-effects. The dose of oral anticoagulant drugs may need to be altered.

ethinyloestradiol continued

Pregnancy,
Breastfeeding

Combined oral contraceptive pills have not been shown to cause problems with pregnancy while they are being used, though they should be stopped before attempting to fall pregnant. The 'pill' decreases the supply of breastmilk and is not recommended for use while breastfeeding.

Special Features,
Comments

Serious problems can occur with the the use of oestrogens. These include blood clots affecting the brain, lungs and heart, gall bladder disease and possibly increase the risk of cancer of the uterus (if used alone as hormone replacement). Most women do not develop these problems. A regular review of treatment is important, as for any long term medication.

ethosuximide

Trade Names	Emeside, Zarontin
How Available	tablet, syrup
Drug Group	Anticonvulsant (drug used in epilepsy)
Prescription	Yes

Major Uses

This medication is used in the treatment of one form of epilepsy known as absence seizures (petit mal). It is generally not effective in other types of seizures.

How it Works

Ethosuximide acts on the cerebral cortex and dampens down electrical activity coming from the motor section of the brain as well as making the brain less sensitive to electrical stimuli which could cause epilepsy.

Usual Dosage

The dose varies according to the response. A low dose 500mg is the usual initial dose in adults. It is increased slowly till the optimum response is achieved. A maximum dose of 1500mg per day is usual. In children the dose depends on age and weight.

Common Side-Effects

Loss of appetite, nausea, abdominal cramps, drowsiness and dizziness are possible common side-effects. Rashes, other gastro-intestinal problems, headache and hiccoughs may occur. Rarely, blood cell production may be interfered with, a potential worry as the drug is intended for long-term use.

Actions with other Drugs

Any medication which can cause sedation will add to the sedative side-effects of ethosuximide. Sleep drugs, antihistamines, benzodiazepines, antidepressants, strong analgesics and major tranquillisers will display this additive effect as will alcohol. Carbamazepine may decrease the levels of ethosuximide in the blood, while phenytoin and sodium valproate may increase it.

Pregnancy, Breastfeeding

Women who use anticonvulsant drugs during pregnancy have an increased chance of having birth defects. The chance is about three times normal. In many cases, there is no alternative but to use anticonvulsants. The potential problems to mother and baby of uncontrolled fitting during pregnancy outweigh the possibility of having an abnormal child. The drug is passed into breastmilk and safety in nursed infants has not been proven.

Special Features, Comments

Due to the sedative effects of the drug, driving and hazardous work should be undertaken with caution.

famotidine

Trade Names	Pepcid
How Available	tablet
Drug Group	Anti-ulcer drug
Prescription	Yes
Major Uses	Famotidine is used for the treatment of ulcers in the stomach and duodenum. Following healing of an ulcer, famotidine is often continued for a longer period to prevent recurrence. It can also be used to decrease the inflammation caused by stomach acid in the esophagus (reflux oesophagitis).
How it Works	Famotidine is a drug in the class called H2 receptor antagonists. This medication blocks the action of histamine on the cells which produce acid in the stomach. The result is a very large drop in the amount of acid produced. This reduction leads to a decrease in inflammation of the linings of the oesophagus, stomach and duodenum, thus e.g. allowing the healing of an ulcer.
Usual Dosage	40mg at night is the usual adult dose for the treatment of peptic ulcer. A maintenance dose of 20mg at night is then used to prevent recurrence of ulcers. The medication is rarely used in children.
Common Side-Effects	Headache, constipation, dizziness and nausea are possible, but unlikely side-effects. Dry mouth and a rash may occur.
Actions with other Drugs	Unlike cimetidine (another H2 antagonist), famotidine has no known substantial interactions with other drugs.
Pregnancy, Breastfeeding	Though no known problems have been established, famotidine is not recommended for use in pregnancy or breastfeeding. It is used only if absolutely necessary.
Special Features, Comments	Alcohol and cigarettes can prevent ulcer healing, so they should not be taken with famotidine. This medication should be used with caution in people with impaired kidney function.

felodipine

Trade Names	Plendil
How Available	tablet, slow release tablet
Drug Group	Calcium channel blocker
Prescription	Yes

Major Uses
Felodipine is used in the treatment of raised blood pressure. Calcium channel blockers are thought to prevent the flow of calcium in the walls of smooth muscle cells which line small arteries. This decreases blood pressure, increases flow through the arteries and prevents spasm of the walls of arteries (which occurs in the heart in some attacks of angina).

How it Works
5-10mg per day is the usual adult dose of felodipine. It is not generally used in children.

Usual Dosage
Flushing, headaches, ankle swelling, dizziness and tiredness are all common side-effects with this medication. They usually occur at the start of treatment and disappear or decrease with time. Other side-effects are possible, but much less common.

Common Side-Effects
Felodipine increases the effects of drugs which lower blood pressure. Beta-blocker medications can act at a similar place in the heart conduction system to lead to a serious slowing of heart rate. Interestingly, the level of felodipine in the blood is increased when taken with grapefruit juice. This is thought to be due to a component unique to grapefruit, as it does not occur with other citrus fruits.

Actions with other Drugs
Medications which may decrease the contraction power of the heart muscle should be used with caution with this drug. Digoxin levels can be increased with felodipine. Cimetidine may increase the level of felodipine in the blood.

Pregnancy, Breastfeeding
Felodipine should not be used in women who are pregnant or attempting to fall pregnant as theoretically it has the potential to cause birth defects. It is generally not recommended in breastfeeding.

Special Features, Comments
Felodipine should be used cautiously in people with poor cardiac function e.g. severe heart failure. It may make this problem worse. Alcohol may accentuate the blood pressure lowering properties of the drug and may cause more side-effects.

fenfluramine

Trade Names	Ponderax
How Available	tablet, capsule
Drug Group	Drug for weight loss
Prescription	Yes
Major Uses	Fenfluramine is used to achieve weight loss as an adjunct to diet. It has been used in overweight people who have diabetes or raised blood pressure.
How it Works	This drug works on areas of the brain responsible for appetite. This reduces food intake and thus weight.
Usual Dosage	One capsule 60mg daily.
Common Side-Effects	Diarrhoea, sedation, sleep disturbances, giddiness and lowered blood pressure are possible side-effects. Other side-effects are much less common.
Actions with other Drugs	Fenfluramine should not be given with other appetite suppressing drugs. A reduction in the dose of fenfluramine may cause depression or reduce the effect of anti-depressants.
Pregnancy, Breastfeeding	This medication is not recommended for use in pregnant women or women who are breastfeeding.
Special Features, Comments	Treatment is usually only for three continuous months. Treatment will only be effective if accompanied by a decrease in calorie intake. Long-term weight reduction will only occur if patterns of food use change.

finasteride

Trade Names	Proscar
How Available	tablet
Drug Group	5 alpha-reductase inhibitor
Prescription	Yes
Major Uses	This drug is used for the treatment of a specific enlargement of the prostate gland in men called benign prostatic hypertrophy (BPH).
How it Works	Finasteride is the first of a new class of medications. It selectively blocks the metabolism of testosterone into the metabolically more active di-hydro testosterone (DHT). DHT is necessary for the development of BPH. The net result is a decrease in the volume of the prostate gland and an improvement in the flow of urine. The effects of finasteride are cumulative and the reduction of prostate volume in BPH takes place over a period of some months. Finasteride should be continued if this effect is to be maintained.
Usual Dosage	One tablet (5mg) per day is the recommended dose. The medication is not recommended for use in children.
Common Side-Effects	Impotence, decreased libido and decreased volume of ejaculate are the most commonly reported side-effects. Other problems appear to be much less likely.
Actions with other Drugs	Few drug interactions of clinical significance have been identified. It may speed up the metabolism of theophylline.
Pregnancy, Breastfeeding	Finasteride is not intended for use in women. In pregnant women there are serious potential side-effects to the development of the male foetus, and it is important that women who are pregnant or planning to become pregnant do not handle the crushed tablets of finasteride.
Special Features, Comments	Finasteride causes a reduction in the blood level of a substance called PSA (prostate specific antigen). This test is used as an aid to the diagnosis of prostate cancer. It is possible that this effect could delay the diagnosis of prostate cancer, though this has not been shown in studies. PSA tests and prostate gland examinations are usually performed before finasteride therapy is commenced.

flucloxacillin

Trade Names	Floxapen, Flucloxacillin, Magnapen, Stafoxil
How Available	capsule, syrup, injection
Drug Group	Penicillin antibiotic
Prescription	Yes
Major Uses	Flucloxacillin is used in a number of infections, most commonly against staphylococcal organisms. Such infections occur most commonly in the skin, soft tissue, burns and wounds. Less often they occur in bone and other organs.
How it Works	This antibiotic prevents the cell wall of the bacteria from being formed, thus killing the organism. Unlike some other types of penicillin, flucloxacillin is generally not broken down by enzymes produced by some staphylococcal bacteria.
Usual Dosage	The usual adult dose is 250-500mg every six hours. Higher doses may be necessary for some infections. In children, half the adult dose is given for children 2-10 years, and a quarter of the adult dose for children less than 2. The medication should be given half to one hour before meals.
Common Side-Effects	Nausea, vomiting, diarrhoea and dyspepsia can occur. An allergic rash is a common side-effect as with other types of penicillin. Other side-effects are less likely.
Actions with other Drugs	Probenecid increases the level of flucloxacillin in the blood.
Pregnancy, Breastfeeding	This drug is generally deemed safe to use in pregnancy if it is thought necessary. If use is required in breastfeeding women (it is sometimes used for the treatment of breast infections) then an alternative food supply for the child may be necessary.

fluconazole

Trade Names	Diflucan
How Available	capsule, intravenous solution
Drug Group	Anti-fungal antibiotic
Prescription	Yes
Major Uses	Most commonly, this drug is used as a treatment for vaginal candidiasis (thrush) when local therapy has failed. It is also used for serious fungal infections within the body and for the treatment of fungal infections in people with impaired immunity.
How it Works	Fluconazole works within the fungal cells to interfere with the function of essential processes.
Usual Dosage	The usual dose for treating vaginal candidiasis is a single 150mg capsule. For other conditions, the dose and length of treatment varies according to the nature of the illness. It is not generally recommended for use in children.
Common Side-Effects	If fluconazole is used for more than seven days nausea, vomiting, skin rash, headache, abdominal pain and diarrhoea are the commonest side-effects. Abnormalities in liver function may occur.
Actions with other Drugs	Fluconazole may increase the effect of warfarin, phenytoin, theophylline and cyclosporin. It reduces the metabolism of some oral drugs used in the treatment of diabetes and may lead to increased blood glucose.
Pregnancy, Breastfeeding	Use in pregnancy should be avoided, unless absolutely necessary. It is not recommended for use in nursing mothers.
Special Features, Comments	In people taking fluconazole for extended periods, periodic blood tests are necessary to monitor liver function.

flunisolide

Trade Names	Syntaris
How Available	Nasal Spray
Drug Group	Cortico-steroid
Prescription	Yes
Major Uses	This drug is used for the prevention and treatment of allergic rhinitis (hay fever).
How it Works	The exact way in which cortico-steroids work on the tissue lining the nose is unknown, but it certainly dampens down many of the inflammatory processes in the cells of the nasal passages.
Usual Dosage	Two sprays in each nostril twice to three times daily is the usual adult dose. Half this dose is recommended for children, though the medication is not recommended for children less than six.
Common Side-Effects	Nasal burning and stinging, nasal dryness, irritation and congestion, nose bleeds and thrush affecting the nose are the commonest side-effects. Other problems are much less likely.
Actions with other Drugs	No significant interactions are known, however the side-effects recorded above could be made more common if flunisolide is used with other nasal medications.
Pregnancy, Breastfeeding	It is not recommended that flunisolide be given to pregnant or breastfeeding women.
Special Features, Comments	Therapy with local steroids may mask early signs of infection. Patients are often advised to discontinue treatment after six months of therapy to assess the effect on the underlying problem.

flunitrazepam

Trade Names	Rohypnol
How Available	tablet
Drug Group	Benzodiazepine
Prescription	Yes

Major Uses　　Flunitrazepam is a strong and very quickly acting medication used to induce sleep. It is usually reserved for use with severe insomnia.

How it Works　　The exact action of this drug and other drugs in the benzodiazepine group is not known. It works on the central nervous system.

Usual Dosage　　0.5mg to 1mg in the evening on going to bed.

Common Side-Effects　　Sleepiness, a hangover type feeling, listlessness and drowsiness are the commonest side-effects with flunitrazepam treatment. Confusion and amnesia are less common, but can occur for a prolonged period after the medication is given. These effects are more likely in the elderly.

Actions with other Drugs　　Any medication which can cause sedation will add to the sedative side-effects of flunitrazepam. Sleep drugs, antihistamines, antidepressants, strong analgesics and major tranquillisers will display this additive effect. Alcohol should not be used at the same time as flunitrazepam.

Pregnancy, Breastfeeding　　This medication is not recommended in pregnancy or breastfeeding. An infant can develop withdrawal symptoms if the drug is used up to the time of delivery, and it can pass into breast milk.

Special Features, Comments　　As with other benzodiazepines, there is a potential for dependence with long term use of the medication. Also overdosage can occur. Excessive sleepiness and the inability to arouse a person who has access to flunitrazepam should lead to the suspicion of overdosage. Immediate medical attention is necessary. Alcohol should be avoided with flunitrazepam. Driving and hazardous work situations should be performed with caution.

fluoxetine

Trade Names	Prozac
How Available	tablet
Drug Group	Antidepressant
Prescription	Yes

Major Uses
Fluoxetine is used for the treatment of many types of depression. Although many claims have been made for the drug, such as the enhancement of memory and the prevention of memory loss, the drug is not recommended in this country for any purpose other than the treatment of depression.

How it Works
It is not known exactly how this drug works, but it is presumed that its antidepressant activity is related to its ability to prevent the uptake by parts of the brain of serotonin (a neurotransmitter).

Usual Dosage
20-80mg per day is the usual adult daily dosage range. It is not recommended for use in children

Common Side-Effects
The commonest side-effects requiring cessation of treatment include nervousness, anxiety and insomnia, dizziness, weakness, headache, a rash and itch. There have been many other effects reported, but these are much rarer.

Actions with other Drugs
A severe reaction has been reported in people taking another type of antidepressant drug (the mono-amine oxidase inhibitors) and fluoxetine. They should not be given together nor should either be commenced while there is any residue of the other in the body. Levels of other antidepressants and diazepam may increased by fluoxetine. Levels of lithium may also change. People taking tryptophan as well as fluoxetine may develop restlessness, agitation and abdominal symptoms.

Pregnancy, Breastfeeding
The drug can be used in pregnancy and breastfeeding, if it is thought to be necessary.

Special Features, Comments
As fluoxetine is metabolised by the liver, impaired liver function may affect elimination of the drug. Elderly people may be more affected by the drug. Like all drugs used for depression, overdose can be potentially serious. If additional medication has been taken, then medical advice should be obtained immediately.

fluphenazine

Trade Names	Decazate, Modecate, Moditen, Motipress, Motival
How Available	tablet, injection
Drug Group	Psychiatric drug
Prescription	Yes
Major Uses	Fluphenazine is a major tranquilliser (phenothiazine type) used for treatment of schizophrenia and other psychiatric problems.
How it Works	The phenothiazines have many activities on the brain and the chemicals which transmit messages in the brain. Their major action is probably related to preventing the action of one of these neurotransmitters, dopamine.
Usual Dosage	This varies considerably. Usually a short acting form of the medication is given at the start of treatment, and, if suitable, longer acting injections may be given. The usual maintenance dose orally in adults is 2.5-10mg every six to eight hours. 12.5-50mg is given by injection every week or fortnight.
Common Side-Effects	A wide variety of side-effects can occur. Common ones include dry mouth, blurred vision, drowsiness, sedation, headache, constipation, confusion and movement disorders. These include slow movements and a tremor like Parkinson's disease or longer term problems with involuntary movements. Weight gain may occur.
Actions with other Drugs	Sleep drugs, antihistamines, benzodiazepines, antidepressants, strong analgesics and major tranquillisers add to the sedative effect of fluphenazine as does alcohol. Fluphenazine may decrease the beneficial effects of drugs used for Parkinson's disease. Other drugs which have anticholinergic properties may add to the side-effects of fluphenazine. Medical advice should be sought before taking other medication as further interactions are possible.
Pregnancy, Breastfeeding	After birth, babies of women who have taken fluphenazine may have movement disorders. Fluphenazine is generally not used in pregnancy or breastfeeding, unless absolutely necessary.
Special Features, Comments	If used long term, irreversible movement problems may occur. The medication may need to be stopped before surgery. Driving and hazardous work should be performed with great caution. Alcohol should be avoided. Routine blood tests may need to be performed as liver function can be affected with long term use.

fosinopril

Trade Names	Staril
How Available	tablet
Drug Group	ACE inhibitor (angiotensin converting enzyme inhibitor)
Prescription	Yes
Major Uses	This medication is most commonly used for the long-term treatment of raised blood pressure.
How it Works	Fosinopril works mainly by preventing the action of angiotensin converting enzyme in transforming angiotensin I to angiotensin II. Angiotensin II is a very active substance, so stopping its formation generally leads to a reduction in blood pressure.
Usual Dosage	10-40mg per day as a single dose. This medication has not been proven safe for children, and is not recommended for their use.
Common Side-Effects	Headache, dizziness, fatigue, nausea, vomiting, diarrhoea, abdominal pain and cough are the commonest side-effects and may require cessation of therapy. Other side-effects are much less likely. ACE inhibitors often cause a taste disturbance which subsides after 1-3 months of treatment.
Actions with other Drugs	Excessive lowering of blood pressure may occur in people taking other blood pressure medication, and especially fluid tablets. As ACE inhibitors prevent the loss of potassium, drugs which add or spare potassium are generally not given at the same time. Fosinopril may cause a rise in serum lithium levels. Fosinopril absorption may be affected by the use of antacids.
Pregnancy, Breastfeeding	Fosinopril and other ACE inhibitors are not recommended for use in pregnancy as they may cause birth defects. It is not advised for use by nursing mothers.
Special Features, Comments	ACE inhibitors should be used with caution in people with impaired kidney function and in people with narrowing of their heart valves. Older patients may be more susceptible to the medication. Tests on blood chemistry may be necessary from time to time.

framycetin

Trade Names	Sofradex, Soframycin, Sofra-Tulle
How Available	eye drops, ear drops, ointment, as an addition to sterile gauze
Drug Group	Topical antibiotic
Prescription	Yes
Major Uses	This antibiotic can be used effectively against most bacteria that cause skin, eye and outer ear infections. Due to its toxic effects on the kidney and inner ear, it is not used orally or in any situation where it is absorbed into the body.
How it Works	This medication effectively kills bacteria at low concentrations.
Usual Dosage	Apply to the affected area two to three times per day.
Common Side-Effects	Local allergic problems and rashes can occur. Other problems are rare.
Actions with other Drugs	Nil.
Pregnancy, Breastfeeding	As the medication is not absorbed, no particular problems are expected.

frusemide

Trade Names	Dryptal, Diumide-K Continus, Fru-Co, Frumil, Frusene, Lasikal, Lasilactone, Lasix, Lasoride
How Available	tablet, injection
Drug Group	Loop diuretic (fluid tablet)
Prescription	Yes
Major Uses	Frusemide effectively removes excess fluid from the body. This is most commonly necessary in heart failure, but also in kidney and liver failure. It is also used to lower blood pressure, often combined with other medications.
How it Works	Frusemide inhibits the kidney's ability to concentrate urine. The result is that the kidney produces a far greater quantity of urine.
Usual Dosage	This depends on the nature and severity of the problem treated. The usual starting dose for adults is 40mg per day. This is increased as necessary. It is given in the morning and, if necessary, at midday, to minimise inconvenience to patients. In children weight and age help determine dosage. As the medication depletes the body's potassium store, supplements are given.
Common Side-Effects	Dizziness, tiredness, weakness and muscle cramps are the most common side-effects. The levels of potassium and sodium in the blood can be altered. Blood tests at regular intervals may be necessary. A rash can occur, though more serious allergic problems are unlikely. Ringing in the ears and deafness can occur if very high doses are used. Frusemide may lead to an attack of gout.
Actions with other Drugs	Other fluid tablets can accentuate the potassium losing properties of frusemide. Toxic effects of digoxin are more common if the blood potassium level is low. Some antibiotics and aspirin may cause hearing problems if given in high doses with frusemide.
Pregnancy, Breastfeeding	It is possible that frusemide may cause some problems in the fetus. It is not usually given and may adversely affect some women who have raised blood pressure in pregnancy. The medication may reduce milk supply and pass into breastmilk. It is generally not recommended in breastfeeding.
Special Features, Comments	People with bladder problems may be adversely affected by the increase in urine production. Regular blood samples checking potassium levels may be necessary. Alcohol may lead to dehydration.

gemfibrozil

Trade Names	Lopid
How Available	tablet
Drug Group	Lipid-lowering drug
Prescription	Yes
Major Uses	Gemfibrozil is used to reduce blood cholesterol in various types of conditions in which cholesterol is elevated. The drug is also used in lipid problems associated with diabetes. It is important to remember that all lipid-lowering agents are used as an adjunct to diet therapy.
How it Works	The exact mechanism by which gemfibrozil works is unknown. However, it causes a reduction in two important type of blood fats (very low density lipoproteins and low density lipoproteins). The net effect is to decrease total cholesterol without having an adverse effect on the relatively beneficial high density lipoprotein (HDL) cholesterol.
Usual Dosage	600mg two times per day half an hour before breakfast or the evening meal. It is not recommended for use in children.
Common Side-Effects	Dyspepsia, abdominal pain, diarrhoea, fatigue, nausea and vomiting, rash, vertigo, constipation and headache are the commonest side-effects. Others have been reported, but are less likely.
Actions with other Drugs	Gemfibrozil may make anticoagulant drugs such as warfarin more effective and blood tests need to be monitored more closely if the drugs are used together. A possible rare problem of serious damage to muscles may occur with some other lipid-lowering drugs (HMG CoA reductase inhibitors).
Pregnancy, Breastfeeding	The safe use of the drug in pregnancy and breast feeding has not been established. The drug is generally not recommended for either situation.
Special Features, Comments	Use of gemfibrozil may increase the risk of development of gallstones and gall bladder disease.

glibenclamide

Trade Names	Calabren, Daonil, Euglucon, Semi-Daonil
How Available	tablet
Drug Group	Oral antidiabetic drug (sulphonylurea)
Prescription	Yes

Major Uses

Glibenclamide is only useful in NIDDM (non-insulin dependent diabetes mellitus), if diet alone does not give adequate control. Since it is more active than other sulphonylureas, it is sometimes used if these fail to achieve adequate control.

How it Works

This type of oral antidiabetic drug (sulphonylurea drugs) lowers blood glucose levels by stimulating the pancreas to produce more insulin (the hormone mostly responsible for increasing uptake of glucose into cells). They do not produce more insulin. When using glibenclamide it is vital to follow a diabetic diet.

Usual Dosage

2.5-20mg per day as a single morning dose usual for adults. NIDDM does not occur in children, so glibenclamide is not prescribed.

Common Side-Effects

The most common and most worrying side-effect of oral antidiabetic drugs is that they may lower blood glucose excessively (hypoglycaemia). The warning signs of this are confusion, feeling faint and weak, sweating and tremor. It should be suspected if any of these symptoms develop and requires some immediate carbohydrate treatment e.g. a sweet biscuit or glucose drink. Other side-effects with glibenclamide are nausea and a rash.

Actions with other Drugs

Other drugs given at the same time can lower blood glucose and make hypoglycaemia more likely. These include betablockers, alcohol, other blood glucose lowering agents, aspirin, sulphonamide and tetracycline antibiotics, chloramphenicol and anti-coagulant drugs. Other drugs may decrease the effect of sulphonylureas, including steroids, oestrogens and some fluid tablets.

Pregnancy, Breastfeeding

Control of diabetes in pregnancy is usually achieved with insulin (control is much better), so oral antidiabetic drugs are not used. They are not often used in nursing mothers.

Special Features, Comments

Regular blood and/or urine testing for glucose is necessary. The medication may cause metabolic problems if the body is under severe stress. Overdosage with glibenclamide may lead to unconsciousness and requires immediate medical treatment.

gliclazide

Trade Names	Diamicron
How Available	tablet
Drug Group	Oral antidiabetic drug (sulphonylurea)
Prescription	Yes
Major Uses	Glicazide is only useful in NIDDM (non-insulin dependent diabetes mellitus) if diet alone is inadequate to control blood glucose. It is vital that a diabetic diet is followed, while the medication is used.
How it Works	This type of oral antidiabetic drug (sulphonylurea drugs) lower blood glucose levels by stimulating the pancreas to produce more insulin (the hormone mostly responsible for increasing uptake of glucose into cells). They do not produce more insulin. Glicazide may also work by other means to control blood glucose. It may also have the beneficial effect of reducing blood clotting.
Usual Dosage	40-320mg per day, usually in divided doses. NIDDM does not occur in children, so the medication is not prescribed.
Common Side-Effects	The most common and most worrying side-effect of oral antidiabetic drugs is that they may lower blood glucose excessively (hypoglycaemia). The warning signs of this are confusion, feeling faint and weak, sweating and tremor. It should be suspected if any of these symptoms develop and requires some immediate carbohydrate treatment e.g. a glucose sweet or drink. Other side-effects include nausea, constipation, a rash and altered liver function.
Actions with other Drugs	Other drugs given at the same time can lower blood glucose and make hypoglycaemia more likely. These drugs include alcohol, betablockers, other blood glucose lowering agents, aspirin, cimetidine, sulphonamide and tetracycline antibiotics as well as chloramphenicol and anti-coagulant drugs. Other drugs which decrease the effects of glicazide include steroids and oestrogens.
Pregnancy, Breastfeeding	Control of diabetes in pregnancy is usually achieved with insulin (control is much better), so oral antidiabetic drugs are not used. They are not generally used in nursing mothers.
Special Features, Comments	Regular blood and/or urine testing for glucose is necessary. Medication may cause metabolic problems if the body is under severe stress. Overdosage with glicazide may lead to unconsciousness and requires immediate medical treatment.

glipizide

Trade Names	Glibenese, Minodiab
How Available	tablet
Drug Group	Oral antidiabetic drug (sulphonylurea)
Prescription	Yes
Major Uses	Glipizide is only useful in NIDDM (non-insulin dependent diabetes mellitus) if diet alone cannot give adequate blood glucose control. It is vital that a diabetic diet is followed while the medication is used.
How it Works	This type of oral antidiabetic drug (sulphonylurea drugs) lower blood glucose levels by stimulating the pancreas to produce more insulin (the hormone mostly responsible for increasing uptake of glucose into cells). They do not produce more insulin.
Usual Dosage	2.5-15mg per day, often in divided doses, is usual for adults. NIDDM does not occur in children, so glipizide is not prescribed.
Common Side-Effects	The most common and most worrying side-effect of oral antidiabetic drugs is that they may lower blood glucose excessively (hypoglycaemia). The warning signs of this are confusion, feeling faint and weak, sweating and tremor. While this is rare in long term treatment with glipizide, it should be suspected if any of these symptoms develop and requires immediate carbohydrate treatment with a sweet biscuit or glucose drink. Nausea, vomiting, diarrhoea, constipation and dizziness can all occur.
Actions with other Drugs	Other drugs given at the same time can lower blood glucose and make hypoglycaemia more likely. These drugs include alcohol, betablockers, other blood glucose lowering agents, aspirin, sulphonamide and tetracycline antibiotics as well as chloramphenicol and anti-coagulant drugs. Other drugs may decrease the effect of sulphonylureas including steroids, oestrogens and fluid tablets.
Pregnancy, Breastfeeding	Control of diabetes in pregnancy is usually achieved with insulin (control is much better), so oral antidiabetic drugs are not generally used. They are not often used in nursing mothers.
Special Features, Comments	Regular blood and/or urine testing for glucose is necessary. Glipizide's elimination from the body may be impaired in people with kidney or liver disease. The medication may cause metabolic problems if the body is under severe stress. Overdosage may lead to unconsciousness and requires immediate medical treatment.

glyceryl trinitrate

Trade Names	Coro-Nitro spray, Deponit, GTN, Minitran, Nitrocine, Nitrocontin Continus, Nitrolingual, Nitronal, Percutol, Suscard Buccal, Sustac, Transiderm-Nitro, Tridil
How Available	tablet, continuous release skin patch, ointment, injection
Drug Group	Anti-angina drug
Prescription	Yes, usually
Major Uses	Glyceryl trinitrate is used to prevent and treat angina (a condition in which oxygen supply to the heart muscle is insufficient). It may also be used to treat heart failure after a heart attack and can be used to lower blood pressure during surgery.
How it Works	This medication acts in a number of ways to prevent and treat angina. It reduces the amount of oxygen that the heart needs by decreasing the pressure that the heart pumps against. It also redistributes blood flow within the heart muscle and dilates the arteries leading to the heart muscle.
Usual Dosage	10mg four times per day is the usual oral dose in adults for angina prevention. Glyceryl trinitrate is easily absorbed into the blood from the skin, so sustained release patches and ointment are used. These are applied once or twice per day. To treat an attack of angina, a glyceryl trinitrate tablet which dissolves can be placed under the tongue.
Common Side-Effects	Flushing, dizziness, and headache are all common side-effects and relate directly to the way in which glyceryl trinitrate works. A severe fall in blood pressure and fainting can occur. Side-effects are more common in elderly people. Local irritation to the skin can occur with ointment or the adhesive section of sustained release patches.
Actions with other Drugs	Other blood pressure lowering drugs and alcohol may increase the side-effects of glyceryl trinitrate.
Pregnancy, Breastfeeding	There are very few instances in which this medication would be used in either pregnancy or breastfeeding. Glyceryl trinitrate has not been shown to be safe in either.
Special Features, Comments	The effect of sustained release patches may diminish if used continuously. Often they are only used for twelve to sixteen hours per day. Angina pectoris is a serious medical problem. If an attack does not respond to treatment with this medication in the usual dose, then immediate hospital treatment is vital.

griseofulvin

Trade Names	Fulcin, Grisovin
How Available	tablet
Drug Group	Anti-fungal antibiotic
Prescription	Yes
Major Uses	Griseofulvin is an anti-fungal antibiotic with a broad spectrum of action used to treat fungal infections which are not successfully treated with topical lotions and other preparations. These include fungal infections of nails, areas of thick skin and the scalp.
How it Works	This medication affects the way in which fungal cells divide, preventing them from multiplying effectively.
Usual Dosage	330mg-1g per day in divided doses is the usual adult dose, depending on the condition treated. As the types of fungal infections treated are often resistant to therapy, the medication is often used for weeks or months. The dose is reduced in children according to age and weight.
Common Side-Effects	Headache, tiredness, confusion, nausea, loss of taste and diarrhoea are the most common side-effects. Bone marrow production of blood cells may be impaired if the drug is used long-term. A rash can occur, though other allergic problems are rare.
Actions with other Drugs	Griseofulvin reduces the effect of anti-coagulants and decreases the effect of the oral contraceptive pill.
Pregnancy, Breastfeeding	Griseofulvin has not been established as safe for use in pregnancy or breastfeeding, so it is not generally used in either unless there are very clear benefits outweighing possible problems.
Special Features, Comments	Blood tests are necessary if the drug is used for prolonged periods to detect blood cell problems before they become serious. Alcohol may increase the sedative effects of griseofulvin.

haloperidol

Trade Names	Dozic, Haldol, Haloperidol, Serenace
How Available	tablet, liquid, injection
Drug Group	Anti-psychotic drug (butyrophenone)
Prescription	Yes
Major Uses	Haloperidol is used in the long term treatment of schizophrenia and to reduce aggressive behaviour. It is often used when alcohol withdrawal leads to confusion, hallucinations and aggressive behaviour. The medication can also be used to treat nausea and vomiting associated with advanced cancer.
How it Works	This medication has a number of actions dampening down transmission of impulses from the cortex of the brain to movement and wake centres lower in the brain. The exact way in which the drug works is not known.
Usual Dosage	The dose varies widely depending on the response of the patient and the problem for which it is used. 1-15mg per day is the usual range for long term use, though it may be considerably higher if symptoms are difficult to control. The medication is rarely used in children.
Common Side-Effects	Movement disorders can occur with this drug, some similar to the slow movements of Parkinson's disease. Other movement problems include involuntary movements of the limbs. These may continue after the medication is stopped. Drowsiness and sedation may occur. Dry mouth, blurred vision and difficulty passing urine are possible. Other side-effects include weight gain, dizziness, a rash and restlessness. Confusion may occur, especially in elderly people.
Actions with other Drugs	Any medication which can cause sedation will add to the sedative side-effects of haloperidol. Benzodiazepines, sleep drugs, antihistamines, antidepressants, strong analgesics and major tranquillisers will display this additive effect as will alcohol. Drugs used for the treatment of Parkinson's disease may be affected by haloperidol. Lithium may react adversely with haloperidol. Drugs which cause anti-cholinergic side-effects will add to these adverse effects if used with this medication. In people who are epileptic, it may be necessary to increase the dose of some anti-convulsant medications.

haloperidol continued

Pregnancy, Breastfeeding

There is some evidence that haloperidol may cause fetal abnormalities so it is not generally used in pregnancy, unless absolutely necessary. Safety in breastfeeding has not been proven, so it is not generally recommended.

Special Features, Comments

Long term use of this medication may cause permanent movement disorders. People should be warned that haloperidol may impair mental skills, so that driving and dangerous occupations should be approached cautiously. Alcohol will increase the sedative effects of the drug.

hydrochlorothiazide

Trade Names	Accuretic, Capozide, Carace, Co-Betaloc, Dyazide, Hydromet, Innozide, Kalten, Moducren, Moduret 25, Monozide 10, Secadrex, Sotazide, Tolerzide, Triam-Co, Zestoretic
How Available	tablet
Drug Group	Fluid tablet (thiazide diuretic)
Prescription	Yes
Major Uses	Hydrochlorothiazide is used to lower blood pressure and reduce the build up of fluid that can occur in heart, liver and kidney failure. It can be effective in reducing fluid accumulation prior to menstrual periods. Sometimes, some types of kidney stones will respond to hydrochlorothiazide.
How it Works	Hydrochlorothiazide acts on the kidney to decrease the reabsorption of salts and water.
Usual Dosage	25-50mg daily in the mornings is the usual adult dose, although considerably higher doses can be used if necessary.
Common Side-Effects	Leg cramps can occur as may dizziness and tiredness. Prolonged use can lead to a depletion of potassium. Often a potassium replacement is used at the same time to prevent this potential problem. (Some of the tablets listed above have diuretics other than hydrochlorothiazide in them, which help to conserve potassium.)
Actions with other Drugs	Some anti-inflammatory drugs may reduce the effect of this drug. Digitalis side-effects are more likely due to potassium depletion. Lithium levels can be increased. Alcohol may accentuate the fall in blood pressure that occurs on standing. Other medications which lower blood pressure can cause excessive blood pressure falls.
Pregnancy, Breastfeeding	Diuretics are not generally used to treat raised blood pressure in pregnancy. It may accentuate problems of blood flow to the fetus. Milk supply may diminish when it is used by breastfeeding mothers, so it is not commonly used.
Special Features, Comments	Blood tests may be necessary from time to time to check on potassium levels. Long-term treatment may impair glucose tolerance mimicking diabetes, though stopping the drug reverses this. An increase in uric acid level may occur and lead to gout. In severe liver disease this medication may be dangerous. Thiazide diuretics may increase blood cholesterol levels.

hydrocortisone

Trade Names: Cobadex, Colifoam, Corlan, Daktacort, Dioderm, Econacort, Efcortelan, Epifoam, Eurax-hydrocortisone, Fucidin H, Gentisone HC, Gregoderm, Hydrocal, Hydrocortistab, Hydrocortisyl, Hydrocortone, Mildison Lipocream, Neo-Cortef, Otosporin, Perinal, Proctofoam HC

How Available: tablet, injection, suppository, ointment, ear drops, eye drops

Drug Group: Corticosteroid

Prescription: Yes (in most cases. Lower strength ointments can be obtained without prescription).

Major Uses: This medication is used in a number of situations, most commonly to treat inflammation and allergic reactions in the skin, eye and ear. It can be used to reduce the inflammation of haemorrhoids. Tablets can be taken orally if the body is deficient in naturally produced corticosteroids (which are vital for proper functioning) or if extra corticosteroids are necessary.

How it Works: Hydrocortisone is very similar to a hormone produced by the body and it replaces this natural substance when taken by mouth. The exact way that it reduces inflammation in the skin and other sites is unknown, though one important effect is preventing cells which cause inflammation from arriving at the inflamed tissue.

Usual Dosage: This varies according to the nature and severity of the condition being treated. Topical preparations are used two to three times per day.

Common Side-Effects: All corticosteroids can produce a similar range of side-effects. If taken orally these include indigestion, nausea, weight gain, acne, weakness and thin bones. Peptic ulcer may occur. These side-effects usually occur with long-term treatment. Topical preparations can lead to thinning of the skin if used continuously. A rash may also occur. Use of topical medications does not cause side-effects within the body.

continued over page...

hydrocortisone continued

Pregnancy, Breastfeeding

Corticosteroids, given orally, may increase the frequency of birth defects and decrease the baby's weight. However, late in pregnancy, if a premature delivery is anticipated, they may be beneficial with a short course of hydrocortisone often given to prevent respiratory distress in the baby. Otherwise, hydrocortisone is used only if absolutely necessary. It is generally avoided in breastfeeding as it does pass into breastmilk.

Special Features, Comments

Blood tests at regular intervals may be necessary. Checks should be made from time to time to ensure that glaucoma (raised eye pressure) and diabetes are not present. Alcohol may increase the chance of peptic ulcer if taken with oral hydrocortisone.

hyoscine

Trade Names	Buscopan, Scopoderm
How Available	tablet, injection, sustained release skin patch, liquid, eye drops
Drug Group	Anti-cholinergic drug
Prescription	Yes (No for some motion sickness preparations)
Major Uses	The commonest use of this medication is to help prevent motion sickness. It can also be used to prevent spasm of the wall of the gut and so stop the pain of 'irritable bowel'. It is also useful for pain due to kidney stones. Frequently, it is given as part of an injection before surgery. Eye drops are used to dilate the pupil and allow better examination of the eye.
How it Works	This drug acts to dampen down one arm of the nervous system (the parasympathetic nervous system). All of its actions and side-effects are a result of this ability to block transmission in these nerves.
Usual Dosage	Doses vary according to the nature and severity of the condition treated and also the other medications used with hyoscine (if used in combination). Normally the tablets are used 3-4 times daily. Hyoscine should be given 30 to 60 minutes before travel to prevent motion sickness. Transdermal patches are used before and during travel.
Common Side-Effects	Tiredness, drowsiness, dry mouth, difficulty passing urine, blurred vision and constipation are all common side-effects. Other side-effects are much less common.
Actions with other Drugs	Any medication which can cause sedation will add to the sedative side-effects of hyoscine. Sleep drugs, antihistamines, antidepressants, strong analgesics, benzodiazepines and major tranquillisers will display this additive effect as will alcohol.
Pregnancy, Breastfeeding	Though no specific problems have been recorded, this medication is not generally recommended for use in pregnancy or breastfeeding.
Special Features, Comments	People should be warned that hyoscine may impair mental skills, so that driving and hazardous occupations should be approached cautiously. This is particularly vital as the medication is used to prevent travel sickness. Alcohol will add to this sedative effect.

ibuprofen

Trade Names	Apsifen, Brufen, Codafen Continus (with codeine), Fenbid Spansule, Ibugel, Junifen, Lidifen, Motrin, Nurofen, Proflex
How Available	tablet, capsule, liquid, cream
Drug Group	NSAID (non-steroidal anti-inflammatory drug)
Prescription	Yes, usually
Major Uses	Ibuprofen is a NSAID which is used in a variety of complaints including many types of arthritis and the pain, and stiffness associated with short and long-term inflammation of joints and soft tissues. Ibuprofen can be used to treat pain associated with menstrual periods and common colds, headaches and dental pain.
How it Works	This drug inhibits the formation of prostaglandins which act on local tissues to produce pain and inflammation.
Usual Dosage	200mg-2.4g daily depending on the type and severity of the condition treated. It is not recommended for use in children.
Common Side-Effects	All NSAIDs produce gastro-intestinal symptoms to some degree. These most commonly are nausea, vomiting, upper abdominal pain and heartburn. Occasionally, an ulcer or bleeding from the stomach may occur, especially in older people or when therapy is for an extended time. Other side-effects include rash, ringing in the ears and swollen ankles due to fluid retention. To avoid many of these side-effects NSAIDs should only be taken after food.
Actions with other Drugs	Use of this drug with aspirin or steroids may increase the chances of peptic ulcer and bleeding. It should not be used by people with peptic ulcers and only with caution by people with a history of them. This medication may raise the level of digoxin and lithium in the blood. The effect of blood pressure and fluid tablets may be reduced. It may interfere with the effect of anti-coagulant medications.
Pregnancy, Breastfeeding	Ibuprofen may cause some fetal abnormalities early in pregnancy and may also interfere with fetal blood circulation in the heart late in pregnancy. Thus it is not recommended in pregnancy. It has not been shown to cross over to the infant in breast milk, but its use in breastfeeding should be discussed with your doctor.
Special Features, Comments	Should be given with caution to people with impaired liver, kidney or heart function. Alcohol will increase the irritation of the stomach caused by ibuprofen. The medication may interfere with clotting and this should be considered before surgery or dental work.

idoxuridine

Trade Names	Herpid, Virudox, Iduridin
How Available	ointment, drops
Drug Group	Antiviral antibiotic
Prescription	No
Major Uses	Idoxuridine is an antibiotic effective against the herpes simplex virus. It can be used in topical preparations in herpes infections of the lips and eyes. There is no oral form of the drug.
How it Works	This medication resembles one of the building blocks of the genetic material of some viruses (thymidine). Idoxuridine is incorporated into the gene, but this makes the gene less stable and more likely to break down during virus multiplication.
Usual Dosage	Apply every two to three hours throughout the day.
Common Side-Effects	Skin and eye inflammation can occur as well as local allergies. Blurred vision and excessive reaction to light may also be side-effects.
Actions with other Drugs	Some other eye preparations may make eye inflammation more likely if used at the same time as idoxuridine.
Pregnancy, Breastfeeding	No known problems.

imipramine

Trade Names	Tofranil
How Available	tablet, syrup
Drug Group	Tricyclic antidepressant
Prescription	Yes
Major Uses	This medication is used for the treatment of depression. Its sedative effects are less than some other drugs in the group and it is useful if the depressed person is withdrawn. Imipramine is also sometimes used in children for bed-wetting and sometimes for long-term pain. The antidepressant effects start after two to three weeks.
How it Works	The exact mode of action of this group of drugs on the central nervous system is not known.
Usual Dosage	75-200mg daily, usually in a single dose at night. For bed-wetting in children 20-100mg is usual (depending on age and weight).
Common Side-Effects	When imipramine is started or the dose increased some side-effects are common. They include drowsiness, dry mouth, sweating, blurred vision, constipation and difficulty passing urine.
Actions with other Drugs	Sleep drugs, antihistamines, other antidepressants, strong analgesics, benzodiazepines and major tranquillisers add to the sedative effects of imipramine. Imipramine and other tricyclic anti-depressants should not be used at the same time as another type of anti-depressant (MAO inhibitors) as occasionally very serious side-effects may occur. Imipramine may reduce the effect of some blood pressure reducing drugs. Smoking and barbiturates can reduce the anti-depressant effect of this drug.
Pregnancy, Breastfeeding	Safe use of this medication in pregnant women has not been established. Its use should be avoided if possible. Nursing mothers should also avoid the drug as it can pass into breast milk.
Special Features, Comments	All tricyclic antidepressants including imipramine can have serious consequences if an overdose is taken as eventually they will have a profound effect on the heart. Dizziness, blurred vision, dry mouth, agitation, convulsions and lack of arousal should give rise to suspicion of overdosage. Immediate medical attention is imperative. Due to its sedative properties it is important not to drive or do dangerous work until the effect of the drug on the individual is established. Alcohol will increase sedation.

indapamide

Trade Names	Natrilix
How Available	tablet
Drug Group	Antihypertensive (blood pressure lowering) drug
Prescription	Yes
Major Uses	Indapamide is used to lower raised blood pressure. It is usually of most value in mild to moderate increases in blood pressure and is often used in combination with other medications.
How it Works	Indapamide causes a dilation of the blood vessels, and this is probably its most important action, though it is also a diuretic (fluid tablet).
Usual Dosage	One tablet (2.5mg) per day is the usual adult dose. This leads to a reduction in blood pressure which may take up to four to six weeks before the maximal reduction in blood pressure is achieved.
Common Side-Effects	Weakness, dizziness, headache, muscle cramps and nausea can occur, though the medication is generally well tolerated. A lowering of blood potassium levels may occur. Other side-effects are possible but rare.
Action with other Drugs	Indapamide should not be used with other diuretics as this may cause problems with potassium and sodium as well as perhaps causing gout. It may increase the level of lithium in the blood. Other blood pressure lowering medications will add to the effect of indapamide.
Pregnancy, Breastfeeding	Indapamide is not recommended for use either in pregnancy or breastfeeding, though no specific problems have been demonstrated in either.
Special Features, Comments	Blood tests should be performed at regular intervals to check blood potassium levels. Care should be taken in using indapamide in people with severe kidney disease as it may impair function further. Alcohol may increase the blood pressure lowering effect of indapamide.

indomethacin

Trade Names	Flexin Continus, Imbrilon, Indocid, Indolar, Indomod
How Available	tablet, liquid, topical spray, suppository, injection
Drug Group	NSAID (non-steroidal anti-inflammatory drug)
Prescription	Yes
Major Uses	Indomethacin is a very effective NSAID which has been used for many years for a variety of complaints including many types of arthritis and the pain and stiffness associated with inflammation of joints and soft tissues. It is useful in gout, bursitis and inflammation in and around tendons. It can be used for the treatment of menstrual pain.
How it Works	This drug prevents the formulation of substances (prostaglandins) which act on local tissues to produce pain and inflammation.
Usual Dosage	50-200mg per day, depending on the severity and nature of the condition treated. It is not recommended for use in children, although it is sometimes used in juvenile rheumatoid arthritis.
Common Side-Effects	All NSAIDs produce gastro-intestinal symptoms but these are more often seen with indomethacin. These most commonly are nausea, vomiting, upper abdominal pain and heartburn. Diarrhoea is less frequent. Headache, dizziness and lightheadedness can occur. Occasionally an ulcer or bleeding from the stomach may occur. Indomethacin can sometimes prevent normal blood cells from forming. There are many other possible but rare side-effects which can occur. Suppositories can give rectal discomfort.
Actions with other Drugs	Use of this drug with aspirin or steroids may increase the chances of peptic ulcer and bleeding. This medication may raise the level of digoxin or lithium in the blood. The effect of blood pressure and fluid tablets (diuretics) may be reduced. It may interfere with the effect of anti-coagulant medications. Levels of probenecid in the blood may be raised with indomethacin.

indomethacin continued

Pregnancy, Breastfeeding   Indomethacin may cause some fetal abnormalities early in pregnancy and may also interfere with fetal blood circulation in the heart late in pregnancy. Thus it is not recommended in pregnancy. It has not been shown to cross over to the infant in breast milk, so its use in breastfeeding should be discussed with your doctor.

Special Features,   This medication should be given with caution in people with impaired liver or kidney function or in people with heart failure. Alcohol will increase the irritation of the stomach caused by indomethacin. This drug should not be used in people with a history of peptic ulcers. The medication may interfere with clotting and this should be considered before surgery or dental work.

insulin

Trade Names Human Actrapid, Human Actraphene, Human Initard, Human Insulatard, Human Mixtard, Human Monotard, Human Protaphane, Human Ultratard, Human Velosulin, Humulin, Humulin Lente, Humulin M, Humulin S, Humulin Zn, Hypurin Isophane, Hypurin Lente, Hypurin Neutral, Protamine Zinc

How Available injection

Drug Group Diabetes drug

Prescription Yes

Major Uses Insulin is used to treat diabetes mellitus. It can be used in people who produce no insulin of their own or in people whose insulin supply is inadequate to control their blood glucose. Insulin must be used together with an effective diabetic diet to ensure adequate control of blood glucose.

How it Works Insulin is normally produced by cells of the pancreas gland in the body. Insulin acts on liver, muscle and fat cells to increase the uptake of glucose into these cells, to allow them to function normally, and maintain the blood glucose at or near normal limits.

Usual Dosage A wide variety of insulins are available. These come from animals (beef, pork insulins) and now they are also made synthetically using bacteria to produce exactly the same molecule as human insulin. The dose of insulin is tailored to each individual and depends on the type of diabetes, type of insulin, age, weight, activity, diet and many other factors. Most commonly at present, two doses of either one or more insulins (drawn into the same syringe) is given both morning and evening.

Common Side-Effects The most worrying side-effect with insulin use is the production of low blood glucose (hypoglycaemia). The symptoms of this are confusion, sweating, weakness and tremor. If it is suspected then carbohydrate (e.g. a glucose sweet, or biscuit) should be eaten immediately to prevent a more serious fall in blood glucose. Irritation around the site of the injection and local allergy can occur. Other allergic problems are possible.

Actions with other Drugs The following drugs increase blood glucose and thus decrease the effect of insulin: corticosteroids, most diuretics, oral contraceptive pills and thyroxine. Some drugs have the opposite effect and a decrease in the dose of insulin may be necessary. These include *insulin continued*

anabolic steroids, some antidepressants and aspirin in large doses. Betablockers may mask the symptoms of a fall in blood glucose.

Pregnancy, Breastfeeding

Insulin is the usual medication used for the control of diabetes in pregnancy. The insulin needs of women change throughout pregnancy and very close monitoring of blood glucose during pregnancy is vital if the potentially serious problems of poorly controlled diabetes are to be avoided. Insulin does not pass into breastmilk, and there are no special problems with its use in breastfeeding.

Special Features, Comments

Regular monitoring of glucose in the blood and possibly urine are necessary for good control of diabetes. In times of physical stress, and before and after surgery, or with illness, the dose of insulin may need considerable adjustment. Alcohol can interfere with diabetic control and should be avoided with insulin. Diabetes is a long term medical problem and close liaison with a doctor is necessary to obtain the best control and avoid problems.

ipratropium

Trade Names	Atrovent, Duovent, Rinatec,
How Available	puffer, nebuliser solution, nasal spray
Drug Group	Bronchodilator
Prescription	Yes

Major Uses

Ipratropium is used in the treatment of asthma and allergic rhinitis (hay fever). It is also useful in treating breathlessness associated with chronic bronchitis and emphysema. People who have heart problems will have fewer problems with this drug than with stimulant drugs e.g. salbutamol and terbutaline. The two types of drugs can be effectively used together.

How it Works

This medication does not act in the same way as other bronchodilators. While these other drugs stimulate receptors on airway smooth muscle cells, ipratropium blocks the action of another arm of the nervous system (the anti-cholinergic nervous system). The end result is a relaxation of the bronchial smooth muscle and easier passage of air through the small airways.

Usual Dosage

Two puffs three to four times per day is the normal adult dose. The nasal spray is given in a similar dose. In children the doses given depend on age and weight.

Common Side-Effects

Dry mouth is a possible side-effect. Blurred vision can occur if the medication is not handled properly and comes into contact with the eye. Other side-effects are rare in normal dosages. Local nasal irritation, dry nose and stuffiness may occur with the nasal spray.

Actions with other Drugs

No interactions are known to occur with ipratropium.

Pregnancy, Breastfeeding

Although no definite problems have been established, care is advised in pregnancy and the medication used only if thought necessary. The medication should be used by nursing mothers only if potential benefits outweigh possible risks.

Special Features, Comments

If the usual dose of the medication does not relieve breathlessness as expected, then medical advice should be promptly sought.

iron

Trade Names   Bioglan Hemofactor, Calvita, Clements Iron, Fefol, Fergon, Ferro-
                        Gradumet, Ferrum-H, Fespan, FGF, Iron Compound

How Available   tablet, injection, solution

Drug Group   Essential mineral

Prescription   No

Major Uses   Iron is used for the treatment of iron deficiency, iron deficiency
                        anaemia and to prevent iron deficiency from occurring in pregnancy
                        and breastfeeding.

How it Works   Iron is essential for the formation of haemoglobin. Most cells in the
                        body require small amounts of iron also, and some tissues (e.g.
                        muscle) require much larger amounts.

Usual Dosage   The usual dose for use in pregnancy is about 100mg of elemental
                        iron per day. Much higher doses can be given orally for iron
                        deficiency and, if necessary, injections of iron may be used.

**Common
Side-Effects**   Nausea and constipation are possible side-effects of iron treatment.
                        As much of the iron is not absorbed, the colour of bowel movements
                        will be darker. An allergic rash may occur with oral tablets, but more
                        serious allergic problems can occur with injected forms. Skin
                        staining can occur around the injection site.

**Actions with other
Drugs**   Some medications such as tetracycline antibiotics, cholestyramine
                        and antacids can interfere with absorption of iron. Vitamin C taken
                        at the same time may increase absorption.

**Pregnancy,
Breastfeeding**   Iron supplements have long been used in pregnancy and are
                        considered safe for use in pregnancy and breastfeeding.

**Special Features,
Comments**   While iron tablets are generally safe, a large dose taken at one time
                        can lead to very serious problems. It is important to keep the
                        medication in a safe place to avoid accidental overdose by children.
                        Lethargy, vomiting, diarrhoea and collapse can all be signs of
                        overdosage. Immediate medical attention is vital.

isosorbide dinitrate

Trade Names	Cedocard, Imtack, Isoket, Isordil, Sorbichew, Sorbid SA, Sorbitrate, Soni-Slo
How Available	tablet, slow release tablet
Drug Group	Anti-angina drug
Prescription	Yes
Major Uses	Isosorbide dinitrate is used to prevent and treat angina (a condition in which insufficient oxygen is supplied to the heart muscle). It may also be used to treat heart failure after a heart attack.
How it Works	Isosorbide dinitrate acts in a number of ways to prevent and treat angina. It reduces the amount of oxygen that the heart needs by decreasing the pressure that the heart pumps against. It also redistributes blood flow within the heart muscle and dilates the arteries thereby allowing the heart muscle to receive more oxygen.
Usual Dosage	Isosorbide dinitrate can be given under the tongue for rapid absorption to alleviate an attack of angina. The usual dose for this is 5-10mg. Higher doses, 10-30mg four times daily, or a single slow release tablet can be given orally to help prevent angina attacks. The drug is not usually prescribed in children.
Common Side-Effects	Flushing, dizziness, and headache are all common side-effects and relate directly to the way in which isosorbide dinitrate works. A severe fall in blood pressure and fainting can occur. Side-effects are more common in elderly people.
Actions with other Drugs	Other blood pressure lowering drugs and alcohol may increase the side-effects of this medication.
Pregnancy, Breastfeeding	There are few instances in which this medication would be used in either pregnancy or breastfeeding. Isosorbide dinitrate has not been shown to be safe in either and is not recommended.
Special Features, Comments	Angina pectoris is a serious medical problem. If an attack does not respond to treatment with this medication in the usual dose, then immediate hospital treatment is vital. The effects of this drug may diminish with time, requiring an increased dose.

isotretinoin

Trade Names	Isotrex, Roaccutane
How Available	tablet, gel
Drug Group	Drug used for acne
Prescription	Yes

Major Uses
Isotretinoin is an effective drug for the treatment of severe, cystic acne. Due to its potential side-effects, it is not used unless the acne has not responded to other more conventional treatments.

How it Works
The exact way in which this medication works is not known. It does however decrease the function of sebaceous glands in the skin, thus decreasing oil formation within the skin.

Usual Dosage
Up to 30-70mg daily is the average dose. The dose is usually assessed on the basis of the weight of the patient. The initial treatment is continued for 2-8 weeks. During the first two weeks of treatment, acne may actually worsen. If isotretinoin is effective, an interval of eight weeks is maintained between first and second courses, as further improvement may occur, even off therapy.

Common Side-Effects
Inflammation of the lips is very common. Dry nose, mouth and skin are also common as are nose bleeds. Muscle pain, headache and impaired vision can occur along with nausea, vomiting and abdominal pain.

Actions with other Drugs
Tetracycline antibiotics (commonly also used in acne) may lead to increased pressure within the brain and headaches, vomiting. They should not be used at the same time as isotretinoin. Vitamin A (to which isotretinoin is related) may increase this medication's side-effects. Any topical preparation which dries the skin (including some acne lotions) can add to the drying effect of isotretinoin.

Pregnancy, Breastfeeding
Isotretinoin is known to cause serious birth defects if used in pregnancy. Not only is it not recommended to take this medication during pregnancy, but effective contraception should be used to prevent possible pregnancy while this medication is being used. Isotretinoin should not be used during breastfeeding.

Special Features, Comments
Blood tests are necessary from time to time to ensure that blood fats and liver function are not impaired by isotretinoin.

ketoconazole

Trade Names	Nizoral
How Available	tablet, shampoo, cream
Drug Group	Anti-fungal antibiotic
Prescription	Yes
Major Uses	Topical ketoconazole is used to treat a wide variety of fungal infections in the skin. Oral ketoconazole is used to treat infections caused by funguses within the body and also skin and nail infections which have not responded to topical treatment. Unusual fungal infections may respond to oral ketoconazole treatment. Dandruff is in part due to a fungal infection in the scalp, this is why it responds to ketoconazole shampoo.
How it Works	This drug acts by altering the composition of the cell membrane of funguses making them less effective barriers.
Usual Dosage	200-400mg per day is the usual adult dosage, depending on the nature and seriousness of the infection. This medication is not generally used in children. The cream is used once to twice daily and the shampoo once daily.
Common Side-Effects	Nausea, vomiting, abdominal pain, rash, headache and dizziness are all possible side-effects with the oral drug. Alterations in liver function can occur with use extended past a few weeks. Other allergic problems are possible. Occasionally breast tenderness can occur in men. Local skin and scalp irritation can occur with the cream and shampoo.
Actions with other Drugs	Antacids, ranitidine and cimetidine may lead to a decrease in blood levels of oral ketoconazole. (This is because stomach acid is required to dissolve the tablet.) Rifampicin (a drug for tuberculosis) decreases the action of ketoconazole. Ketoconazole increases the effect of cyclosporin.
Pregnancy, Breastfeeding	Oral ketoconazole may cause birth defects, so it is not generally prescribed during pregnancy. It is also not used recommended for nursing mothers. Generally, the cream and shampoo are thought to be safe in both pregnancy and breastfeeding.
Special Features, Comments	Blood tests are taken at regular intervals if oral ketoconazole is taken for long periods to detect any liver test abnormalities.

ketoprofen

Trade Names	Alrheumat, Orudis, Oruvail Gel, Oruvail
How Available	tablet, suppository
Drug Group	NSAID (non-steroidal anti-inflammatory drug)
Prescription	Yes
Major Uses	Ketoprofen is a NSAID which is used in a variety of complaints including many types of arthritis and the pain and stiffness associated with inflammation of joints and soft tissues. It can be used for acute arthritis while other medications are taking effect.
How it Works	This drug prevents the action of substances (prostaglandins) which act on local tissues to produce pain and inflammation.
Usual Dosage	For adults, 100-200mg per day in divided doses or a single dose of the slow release medication is usual. It is not recommended for use in children.
Common Side-Effects	All NSAIDs produce gastro-intestinal symptoms to some degree. These most commonly are nausea, vomiting and upper abdominal pain. It is rare, but possible, for ketoprofen to produce an ulcer in the stomach or duodenum and this may bleed. (For this reason any person with a history of ulcer disease should avoid ketoprofen and NSAIDs generally.) Dizziness, rash and breathlessness can occur.
Actions with other Drugs	Use of this drug with aspirin or steroids may increase the chances of peptic ulcer and bleeding. The effect of blood pressure and fluid tablets (diuretics) may be reduced. It may interfere with the effect of anti-coagulant medications. Ketoprofen may decrease the blood glucose of diabetics taking oral glucose lowering agents.
Pregnancy, Breastfeeding	Ketoprofen may interfere with fetal blood circulation in the heart late in pregnancy. Thus it is not recommended in pregnancy. It is not known if ketoprofen crosses over to the infant in breast milk, so its use in breastfeeding should be discussed with your doctor.
Special Features, Comments	This medication should be given with caution in people with impaired liver function or in people with heart failure. It should not be used in people with a history of peptic ulcers. Alcohol will increase the irritation of the stomach caused by ketoprofen. The medication may interfere with clotting and this should be considered before surgery or dental work.

labetalol

Trade Names	Trandate
How Available	tablet
Drug Group	Drug used for blood pressure
Prescription	Yes
Major Uses	Labetalol is used for the treatment of raised blood pressure.
How it Works	This drug blocks beta receptors as do the betablockers. (It is unclear how this action reduces blood pressure.) It also, however, acts on alpha receptors. This action does lead to a fall in blood pressure, but it also means that labetalol has the potential to cause a greater range of side-effects than beta-blockers.
Usual Dosage	100-200mg twice daily is the usual adult dose. Higher doses can also be used.
Common Side-Effects	Dizziness, headache, depressed mood and excessive lowering of blood pressure on standing are common. A rash, nausea and vomiting and difficulty in passing urine are possible.
Actions with other Drugs	Other drugs which dilate blood vessels add to postural lowering of blood pressure with labetalol. Labetalol should be used with caution with clonidine and methyldopa. Calcium antagonists may markedly reduce heart rate if given with labetalol. Cimetidine can increase the blood level of labetalol.
Pregnancy, Breastfeeding	Labetalol has been used for the treatment of raised blood pressure in pregnant women without recognised adverse effects. It can lower the fetal heart rate and blood glucose. It is not recommended for use by nursing mothers.
Special Features, Comments	It can be dangerous to withdraw this drug suddenly as a rapid rise in blood pressure or increase in heart oxygen consumption may occur. People with diseased arteries to the legs may have increased symptoms if labetalol is used. Unstable diabetics should avoid labetalol as it may mask signs of low blood glucose. People with asthma or chronic bronchitis should avoid labetalol. It may make their problems much worse. The drug may need to be stopped before a general anaesthetic is given. An overdose of this medication can be serious and immediate medical attention should be sought. The medication should be used with caution in people with liver disease.

levodopa

Trade Names	Brocadopa, Larodopa, Madopar, Sinemet
How Available	tablet
Drug Group	Drug for Parkinson's disease
Prescription	Yes
Major Uses	Levodopa is used to treat Parkinson's disease (a relatively common problem leading to an inability to move effectively and also a tremor). Parkinson's-like disease, caused by a viral infection to the brain, may also respond to treatment, though Parkinsonism produced by drugs (e.g. haloperidol) responds less well.
How it Works	Levodopa is converted within the brain into a substance known as dopamine. Certain areas of the brain responsible for movement (the basal ganglia) are very rich in dopamine, which helps transmit nervous impulses. The supply of dopamine in the basal ganglia is known to be dramatically reduced in Parkinson's disease. Levodopa helps replenish it.
Usual Dosage	Levodopa treatment is begun at a low dose (250-500mg per day) and increased slowly to achieve maximum relief with minimal side-effects. The drug is generally not prescribed for children.
Common Side-Effects	Levodopa is often given with another medication which prevents the breakdown of the levodopa before it enters the brain. This allows a smaller overall dose of levodopa to be given, which minimises side-effects, most commonly nausea and vomiting. Loss of appetite and constipation are possible. Involuntary movements, tiredness, low blood pressure, confusion and palpitations may occur.
Actions with other Drugs	Some antidepressants interact with levodopa to give a marked rise in blood pressure. Some other drugs used in psychiatry may add to the side-effects of this drug. Medications which lower blood pressure may cause excessive reductions if used with levodopa. Vitamin B6 (pyridoxine) can prevent the drug from being absorbed.
Pregnancy, Breastfeeding	It is unlikely that the drug would be used in women of childbearing age. Levodopa is not recommended in pregnancy. as it inhibits breastfeeding and may cause problems in breast-fed babies.
Special Features, Comments	Regular monitoring of the blood for liver, blood cell and kidney function is necessary as treatment is usually long-term. The effectiveness of levodopa may decline over time.

levonorgestrel

Trade Names	Cyclo-Progynova, Eugynon 30 (with ethinyloestradiol), Logynon ED (with ethinyloestradiol), Microgynon 30 (with ethinyloestradiol), Microval, Neogest, Norgeston, Norplant, Nuvelle, Ovran 30 (with ethinyloestradiol), Ovranette (with ethinyloestradiol), Schering PC4 (with ethinyloestradiol), Trinordiol (with ethinyloestradiol)
How Available	tablet
Drug Group	Oral contraceptive
Prescription	Yes
Major Uses	This medication is similar to a naturally occurring female sex hormone (progesterone). It is used in many types of oral contraceptive pills, either alone (the progesterone only or 'mini-pill') or in combination with oestrogen in the more commonly prescribed combined pill. It is also used in combination with oestrogen in women taking these hormones as a replacement at and after the menopause.
How it Works	If used alone, levonorgestrel may act by changing the nature of the mucus around the cervix, preventing sperm from fertilising the ovum. In combination with oestrogen it prevents the release of hormones which stimulate the ovary, so no ova are released.
Usual Dosage	30 micrograms is the dose of levonorgestrel in progesterone only pills. It is important that the dose be taken at the same time every day to achieve effective contraception. The dose is considerably higher (75-250 micrograms) with the combined pill.
Common Side-Effects	Change in menstrual periods and irregular menstrual bleeding are common side-effects if the medication is used alone. Weight gain and swollen ankles are also common. Nausea and vomiting are possible. Many other side-effects have been reported with this medication when combined with oestrogen. (See ethinyloestradiol.)
Actions with other Drugs	Many antibiotics can interfere with levonorgestrel absorption and cause irregular menstrual bleeding and, possibly, contraceptive failure. Also, this medication can adversely affect the action of blood glucose lowering drugs, some anticonvulsants, blood pressure lowering drugs and anti-coagulants. It is important to let your doctor know if you are taking any other medications.

levonorgestrel continued

Pregnancy,
Breastfeeding

Levonorgestrel is used in women who are breastfeeding and need contraception. Small amounts of levonorgestrel do pass into the breastmilk, but have not been shown to cause problems.

Special Features,
Comments

Most women use levonorgestrel alone and in combination with oestrogen for many years with minimal problems.

lignocaine

Trade Names   Betnovate Rectal, Calgel, Lignostab

How Available   ointment, spray, suppository, injection

Drug Group   Local anaesthetic

Prescription   Yes, in most instances for higher strength formulations. Many combinations are available without a prescription.

Major Uses   Lignocaine is often used in creams and lotions to soothe areas of inflamed skin or, for example, in haemorrhoid preparations to reduce discomfort. It is important to remember that lignocaine does not treat the underlying cause of the problem. Lignocaine is used by doctors to anaesthetise areas prior to surgery, often avoiding the need for a general anaesthetic. The drug can also be used by injection after a heart attack to treat some rhythm disturbances.

How it Works   Lignocaine blocks transmission of electrical impulses along nerves. If it blocks the nerves that detect pain then no sensation of pain is recorded by the brain and none 'felt'.

Usual Dosage   The dosage depends on the type of use to which lignocaine is put and the nature of the problem involved. If used by injection, the total dose used must be strictly controlled, and only administered by health personnel to avoid serious problems.

Common Side-Effects   Local irritation and allergic rashes can occur with the topical preparations. Side-effects of the injected drug include nervousness, dizziness, blurred vision, nausea and vomiting. Allergic reactions can occur, as can heart rhythm disturbances.

Actions with other Drugs   There are no known interactions with local treatments, though caution must be used with injectable forms as a wide variety of other drugs may influence lignocaine and vice versa.

Pregnancy, Breastfeeding   Lignocaine has been used extensively during pregnancy with no ill effects demonstrated, so it used if necessary. Lignocaine does pass into breastmilk, but is unlikely to cause problems.

lindane

Trade Names	Quellada
How Available	lotion, cream, concentrate
Drug Group	Skin parasite treatment
Prescription	No
Major Uses	This medication is used to treat insect parasite infections in the skin, the most common of which is scabies. It can also be used to treat scalp infections.
How it Works	Lindane is readily absorbed through the skin of insects and produces seizures in the insect. Usually a single treatment is adequate.
Usual Dosage	This varies according to the type of preparation used. Follow the instructions for each type of medication. Often a repeat treatment after one week is advised to ensure a cure.
Common Side-Effects	Rash and skin irritation can occur, though they are not common. Accidental ingestion of the medication can cause convulsions, so care must be taken to keep the container in a safe place.
Actions with other Drugs	Nil known.
Pregnancy, Breastfeeding	Lindane may be absorbed through the skin, so it is not generally prescribed for pregnant women or in breastfeeding.

lisinopril

Trade Names	Carace, Carace Plus, Zestoretic, Zestril
How Available	tablet
Drug Group	ACE inhibitor (angiotensin converting enzyme inhibitor)
Prescription	Yes
Major Uses	This medication is most commonly used for the long-term treatment of raised blood pressure. It can also be used in the treatment of heart failure as can some other ACE inhibitors.
How it Works	Lisinopril works mainly by preventing the action of angiotensin converting enzyme in transforming angiotensin I to angiotensin II. Angiotensin II is a very active substance, so stopping its formation generally leads to a reduction in blood pressure. Reduced blood pressure can reduce the workload on the heart and thus improve its function.
Usual Dosage	5-10mg per day as a single dose is usual, but up to 40mg may be required. This medication has not been proven safe for children, and is not recommended for their use.
Common Side-Effects	Dizziness, headache, weakness, chest pain, nausea and vomiting, a cough and a rash are the commonest side-effects. These may require cessation of the therapy. Other side-effects are much less likely. ACE inhibitors often cause a taste disturbance which subsides after 1-3 months of treatment.
Actions with other Drugs	Excessive lowering of blood pressure may occur in people taking other blood pressure medication, and especially fluid tablets. As ACE inhibitors prevent the loss of potassium, drugs which add or spare potassium are generally not given at the same time. Lisinopril may cause a rise in serum lithium levels. Indomethacin may decrease the efficacy of lisinopril.
Pregnancy, Breastfeeding	Lisinopril and other ACE inhibitors are not recommended for use in pregnancy as they may cause birth defects. It is not advised for use by nursing mothers.
Special Features, Comments	ACE inhibitors should be used with caution in people with impaired kidney function and in people with narrowing of their heart valves. Older patients may be more susceptible to the medication. Tests on blood chemistry may be necessary from time to time.

lithium

Trade Names	Camcolit, Efalith, Li-liquid, Liskonum, Litarex, Phasal, Priadel
How Available	tablet
Drug Group	Drug used for manic-depression
Prescription	Yes
Major Uses	Lithium is a metal which has been used to prevent and treat the mania of manic-depressive illness. Manic-depression is a condition in which there are marked swings in mood from extreme excitement (mania) to depression. This drug can also be used to treat and prevent depression.
How it Works	The exact way in which lithium acts to prevent mood swings is unknown. It may have a variety of actions on the central nervous system.
Usual Dosage	The dose of lithium needed to control symptoms and prevent mania depends on the individual, their weight and metabolism. Blood levels of lithium are taken to ensure that the correct dose is given. Maintenance doses are usually 500mg-1g per day.
Common Side-Effects	Nausea, vomiting and diarrhoea are the most common side-effects of the medication. Tiredness, difficulty walking and slurred speech can occur. Blurred vision, a rash and a metallic taste are possible problems. Overdosage should be suspected if frequent urination and drinking or persistent vomiting occurs. Immediate medical attention is essential.
Actions with other Drugs	A wide variety of drugs can interact with lithium. These include betablockers, tetracyclines, benzodiazepines, anticonvulsants and other medications used in psychiatric illnesses. A doctor should be consulted before any other medication is taken.
Pregnancy, Breastfeeding	Lithium is not recommended for use in pregnancy. It can cause birth defects, and also interfere with the function of the thyroid gland in the fetus. It is strongly recommended that lithium be stopped before a planned pregnancy. As lithium can pass into breastmilk, bottle feeding is recommended.
Special Features, Comments	Prolonged use may lead to kidney and thyroid gland problems. Regular blood tests will detect any problems early. Regular assessment of serum lithium levels are necessary.

loperamide

Trade Names	Imodium, Loperagen
How Available	capsule
Drug Group	Antidiarrhoeal drug
Prescription	No

Major Uses

Loperamide is used to treat many types of diarrhoea. It does not prevent the cause of the diarrhoea, but effectively decreases the amount and frequency of bowel actions. It can be used for the same purpose in people with colostomies.

How it Works

Loperamide acts locally on nerve endings in the wall of the large bowel to decrease movement and thus allows a greater uptake of fluid. Unlike other antidiarrhoeal preparations, it does not have an effect on the central nervous system. Also, it is much more effective than other medications.

Usual Dosage

Two capsules (4mg) at the onset of severe diarrhoea, followed by one capsule with each loose bowel movement is usual. The dose of medication for longer term treatment is 2-8mg per day. The side-effects of this medication are more pronounced in children, so it is not recommended for children less than twelve years of age.

Common Side-Effects

Rebound constipation is a common problem with loperamide, because it is so effective. Flatulence, abdominal pain and nausea can occur. Other side-effects such as a rash are possible, but much less common.

Actions with other Drugs

These are uncommon. The action of sedatives and the sedative effect of alcohol may be increased.

Pregnancy, Breastfeeding

Though no specific problems have been proven, loperamide is not recommended in either pregnancy or breastfeeding.

loratadine

Trade Names	Clarityn
How Available	tablet
Drug Group	Anti-histamine (non-sedating)
Prescription	Yes
Major Uses	Loratadine is used to dampen down allergic reactions. It is used in the treatment of hay fever (allergic rhinitis) as well as other allergic conditions.
How it Works	Anti-histamines prevent histamine from reacting with cells and causing local inflammation. (Histamine occurs in some types of white blood cells and cells known as mast cells.) It is long-acting and need only be taken once per day.
Usual Dosage	One tablet (10mg) once per day.
Common Side-Effects	Side-effects are uncommon with loratadine. Unlike some antihistamines, loratadine does not cross into the central nervous system, and this means it does not generally cause drowsiness. Many adverse experiences have been reported, but they are very rare.
Actions with other Drugs	The blood levels of some antihistamines can be prolonged with the use of erythromycin, which theoretically could cause a dangerous cardiac rhythm problem. This effect has not been reported with loratadine.
Pregnancy, Breastfeeding	The safe use of this drug in pregnancy and breast feeding has not been established. It should be used only if the benefits outweigh the risks.
Special Features, Comments	There is no specific interaction with alcohol, unlike with other antihistamines.

lorazepam

Trade Names	Ativan
How Available	tablet
Drug Group	Benzodiazepine
Prescription	Yes

Major Uses
Lorazepam is used for the short-term treatment of anxiety. It is also used in depression if anxiety is a prominent component of the disease, and in some other psychiatric illnesses (such as obsessive-compulsive disorders). It is also usual as a pre-medicant.

How it Works
The exact action of this drug and of other drugs in the benzodiazepine group is not known but it is thought to depress the activity in that part of the brain which controls emotion.

Usual Dosage
2-3mg per day in divided doses. A low dose is usually used first and increased as necessary.

Common Side-Effects
Sedation, dizziness, weakness and tiredness are the most common side-effects and these usually occur at the start of treatment. Disorientation, headache, nausea and rash are much less frequent side-effects. Side-effects are more common in elderly people.

Actions with other Drugs
Any medication which can cause sedation will add to the sedative side-effects of lorazepam. Sleep drugs, antihistamines, antidepressants, strong analgesics, other benzodiazepines and major tranquillisers will display this additive effect as does alcohol.

Pregnancy, Breastfeeding
This medication is not recommended in pregnancy or breastfeeding. An infant can develop withdrawal symptoms if the drug is used up to the time of delivery, and it can pass into breast milk.

Special Features, Comments
As with other benzodiazepines, there is a potential for dependence with long term use of the medication. Overdosage can occur. Excessive sleepiness and the inability to arouse a person who has access to lorazepam should lead to the suspicion of overdosage. Immediate medical attention is necessary. Alcohol should be avoided with lorazepam treatment. Driving and hazardous work should be performed with caution.

magnesium hydroxide

Trade Names	Actonorm, Aludrox, Carbellon, Diovol, Mucaine, Simeco
How Available	tablet, liquid, powder
Drug Group	Antacid
Prescription	No
Major Uses	Magnesium hydroxide is an antacid which effectively neutralises stomach acid. It can ease the discomfort of acid reflux into the oesophagus and will decrease acid irritation of the stomach. It can be used to decrease the pain of peptic ulcers, but does not heal them.
How it Works	Magnesium hydroxide neutralises acid, thus reducing the ability of the gastric juice to cause or aggravate inflammation. It is usually given with an aluminium salt as this counteracts the diarrhoea that magnesium salts cause.
Usual Dosage	One to two tablets or 10-20ml of liquid is the usual dose that adults use.
Common Side-Effects	Diarrhoea is a common occurrence with magnesium salts..Other side-effects are rare.
Actions with other Drugs	The absorption of many drugs can be affected, either increased or decreased, by antacids. These include antibiotics, cimetidine, iron supplements, digoxin and levodopa. It is best that an antacid is taken at least 90 minutes before or after other medications. Some coated tablets may be broken down by magnesium salts and cause stomach irritation.
Pregnancy, Breastfeeding	Magnesium hydroxide is frequently used in pregnancy and no adverse effects have been noticed in the fetus. It is considered safe to use in pregnancy and breastfeeding.
Special Features, Comments	People with impaired kidney function may be more prone to a build up of magnesium in the blood (and aluminium if a combination is used).

mazindol

Trade Names	Not yet available in the UK
How Available	tablet
Drug Group	Drug for weight reduction
Prescription	No
Major Uses	Mazindol is used for weight loss as an adjunct to diet.
How it Works	This medication works on the central nervous system. It affects the re-uptake of a transmitting substance called nor-adrenaline, leading to a reduced sensation of hunger.
Usual Dosage	2mg per day is the average dose in adults.
Common Side-Effects	Lack of sleep, restlessness, agitation, palpitations, raised blood pressure, dry mouth, nausea and vomiting are potential side-effects. Others are much less common.
Actions with other Drugs	This medication can interact with some antidepressant medications. It may decrease the dose of insulin necessary for some diabetics. Mazindol may counteract the effect of blood pressure lowering drugs. It should not be given with other weight control tablets. Mazindol can make the stimulant effects of coffee and nicotine more pronounced.
Pregnancy, Breastfeeding	This medication is not usually recommended for use in pregnancy or breastfeeding.
Special Features, Comments	Treatment is usually for three continuous months. Treatment will only be effective if accompanied by a decrease in dietary intake. Long-term weight reduction occurs only if patterns of food use change. It should not be used in people with raised eye pressure (glaucoma) or in people with a history of agitation or drug abuse. Driving and hazardous work should be undertaken with caution.

mebendazole

Trade Names	Vermox
How Available	tablet, liquid
Drug Group	Anti-helminth (worm) drug
Prescription	No
Major Uses	Mebendazole is effective in treating all common worm infestations in the gastro-intestinal tract. These include threadworm, roundworm, whipworm and hookworm.
How it Works	This medication is thought to work by preventing sources of energy from being utilised within the cell of the parasite, eventually leading to the death of the worm.
Usual Dosage	To eradicate parasites the following dose is usually given: one tablet (100mg) or 5mls of suspension twice a day for three days. Usually this is repeated two to four weeks after the initial course. The same dose is given to children and adults. Mebendazole is not recommended for children less than two years of age.
Common Side-Effects	Mebendazole is generally well tolerated. Diarrhoea, vomiting, abdominal pain are possible side-effects. Itching, headache and dizziness can occur. Liver function can become impaired occasionally.
Actions with other Drugs	Nil known.
Pregnancy, Breastfeeding	Some animal trials suggest that mebendazole may cause birth defects, therefore it is not recommended for use during pregnancy. If necessary while a woman is breastfeeding, then bottle feeding is generally substituted while the drug is taken.

mebeverine

Trade Names	Colofac, Fybogel, Mebeverine
How Available	tablet
Drug Group	Anti-spasm drug
Prescription	Yes
Major Uses	Mebeverine is used to treat irritable bowel syndrome. This is a common problem in the modern community, with a variety of symptoms including abdominal pain, flatulence and bloating.
How it Works	This medication has a number of actions on the smooth muscle lining the wall of the large bowel. The net result is a decrease in the amount and intensity of contractions in the large bowel and a decrease in the pain and other symptoms that the spasm causes.
Usual Dosage	One tablet (135mg) three to four times per day, shortly before food. This medication is not generally prescribed in children.
Common Side-Effects	Indigestion, nausea, heartburn, dizziness and headache are all possible side-effects, though mebeverine is generally well tolerated.
Actions with other Drugs	No known problems.
Pregnancy, Breastfeeding	Even though no particular problems have been demonstrated, mebeverine is not recommended for use in either pregnancy or breastfeeding.
Special Features, Comments	Mebeverine should not be used in people with heart arrhythmias or severe liver or kidney disease. The tablets contain lactose, which may cause abdominal pain in some people.

mebhydrolin

Trade Names	Not yet available in the UK
How Available	tablet
Drug Group	Antihistamine
Prescription	No
Major Uses	Antihistamines are used to treat a variety of allergic problems, including hay fever, allergic conjunctivitis, eczema as well as more serious allergic conditions.
How it Works	Antihistamines prevent histamine from reacting with cells and causing local inflammation. Histamine is a naturally occurring substance present in some white blood cells (mast cells). This prevents allergic reactions from becoming worse. Unlike some more recently released antihistamines, this medication does cross into the brain causing sedation.
Usual Dosage	50-100mg twice daily is the usual adult dose. The dose is reduced for children.
Common Side-Effects	The sedative side-effects of antihistamines are the most prominent. Dry mouth, nose and throat can occur with mebhydrolin. Nausea, vomiting, abdominal pain, diarrhoea and constipation are rare side-effects.
Actions with other Drugs	Any medication which can cause sedation will add to the sedative side-effects of mebhydrolin. Sleep drugs, antihistamines, antidepressants, strong analgesics and major tranquillisers will display this additive effect as will alcohol. Some antidepressants can increase the dry eye and mouth problems of mebhydrolin.
Pregnancy, Breastfeeding	This medication has been used in pregnancy and no adverse problems have been demonstrated to the mother or fetus. It is generally thought safe to take in pregnancy if necessary. The medication is not recommended during breastfeeding.
Special Features, Comments	The medication should be taken cautiously by people with prostate gland problems, diabetes, thyroid disease, heart disease or in whom glaucoma is suspected. Alcohol should be avoided with this medication to avoid excessive sedation. Driving and hazardous work should be undertaken with extreme care.

mefenamic acid

Trade Names	Ponstan
How Available	tablet
Drug Group	NSAID (non-steroidal anti-inflammatory drug)
Prescription	Yes

Major Uses
Mefenamic acid is used in the prevention and treatment of menstrual period pain. It can also be used in the treatment of soft tissue and joint inflammation.

How it Works
This medication works in much the same way as other NSAIDs. It inhibits the action of substances (prostaglandins) which act on local tissues to produce pain and inflammation. Mefenamic acid may also prevent prostaglandins from being produced.

Usual Dosage
500mg three times per day with food is the usual adult dose. Doses in children depend on weight and age.

Common Side-Effects
All NSAIDs produce gastro-intestinal symptoms. These most commonly are nausea, vomiting, upper abdominal pain and heartburn. Diarrhoea is common with mefenamic acid. Headache, dizziness and light-headedness can occur. Occasionally an ulcer or bleeding from the stomach may occur. Drowsiness, blurred vision, ringing in the ears and a rash can occur. Kidney inflammation is possible, but rare.

Actions with other Drugs
Use of this drug with aspirin or steroids may increase the chances of peptic ulcer and bleeding. This medication may raise the level of lithium in the blood. The effect of blood pressure and fluid tablets (diuretics) may be reduced. It may interfere with the effect of anti-coagulant medications. Mefenamic acid may lower blood glucose in people taking oral glucose lowering drugs.

Pregnancy, Breastfeeding
Mefenamic acid has not been proven safe to take in pregnancy. It may cause birth defects. It is not recommended for use in breastfeeding.

Special Features, Comments
This medication should be given with caution in people with impaired liver or kidney function. Alcohol will increase the irritation of the stomach caused by mefenamic acid. It should not be used in people with a history of peptic ulcers. The medication may interfere with clotting and this should be considered before surgery or dental work.

mefloquine

Trade Names	Lariam
How Available	tablet
Drug Group	Anti-malaria drug
Prescription	Yes

Major Uses
Mefloquine is a medication used for treatment and prevention of malaria. It is usually only used for some types of malaria (certain types of falciparum malaria) that cannot be treated or prevented by using safer medications.

How it Works
Unlike other medications used for malaria, mefloquine can kill parasites within red cells.

Usual Dosage
For adults: one tablet per week to begin one week before entering the malaria area and continuing for four weeks after leaving the area is the usual dose to prevent malaria. Six weeks treatment is the minimum. Dosage is less for the prevention of malaria in children. Higher doses are used to treat established malaria infections.

Common Side-Effects
Dizziness, unsteadiness, diarrhoea, loss of appetite and headache are all potential side-effects. Mefloquine may impair liver function.

Actions with other Drugs
Quinine may lead to increased side-effects if taken with mefloquine as they are closely related.

Pregnancy, Breastfeeding
It is considered dangerous to use mefloquine in pregnancy, due to the potential risk of birth defects. Women taking mefloquine should use contraception to avoid falling pregnant for three months following the last dose. Mefloquine does pass into breastmilk, so bottle feeding is preferred while the medication is used.

Special Features, Comments
Patients with liver or kidney or heart disease should avoid mefloquine treatment. Overdosage with mefloquine can lead to serious heart rhythm disturbances. Immediate medical attention is necessary if an overdose is suspected.

metformin

Trade Names	Glucophage
How Available	tablet
Drug Group	Oral antidiabetic drug
Prescription	Yes

Major Uses

Metformin is useful in the treatment of NIDDM (non-insulin dependent diabetes mellitus) if diet alone cannot control blood levels of glucose. It is vital that a diabetic diet is followed, while the medication is used, if it is to be effective. It is often used if other oral antidiabetic drugs are not effective, and because it acts by a different mechanism, can be used at the same time as other agents (sulphonylureas).

How it Works

Unlike sulphonylureas, metformin increases the uptake of glucose into cells. It does this by increasing the activity of insulin on these cells.

Usual Dosage

500mg-1g three times per day is the usual adult dose. The medication is not prescribed in children.

Common Side-Effects

The most common and most worrying side-effect of oral antidiabetic drugs is that they may lower blood glucose excessively (hypoglycaemia). This is less common with metformin, but can occur, especially if used with other glucose lowering drugs. The warning signs of this are confusion, feeling faint and weak, sweating and tremor. Immediate carbohydrate treatment e.g. a sweet biscuit or glucose sweet should be administered. One serious potential problem with metformin is the development of a metabolic problem known as lactic acidosis. Loss of appetite and weight loss are early signs of this problem. Nausea is a relatively common side-effect of metformin.

Actions with other Drugs

Alcohol should be taken sparingly with metformin treatment. Metformin may interact with anti-coagulants. Other drugs which lower blood glucose may add to metformin's action.

Pregnancy, Breastfeeding

Control of diabetes in pregnancy is usually achieved most effectively with insulin, so oral antidiabetic drugs are not used. Metformin can cause birth defects and lactic acidosis in the fetus. It is not recommended for use in breastfeeding women.

Special Features, Comments

Overdosage with metformin may lead to unconsciousness and requires immediate medical treatment.

methadone

Trade Names	Physeptone
How Available	tablet, injection
Drug Group	Narcotic analgesic
Prescription	Yes
Major Uses	Methadone is used for severe pain. It can be used in similar situations that morphine would be used. It may cause less mood change than morphine which may be of benefit to cancer patients. It is used under strict medical supervision in narcotic addicted people in long term treatment programmes.
How it Works	Methadone acts on specific receptors in the central nervous system and other tissues.
Usual Dosage	The dose varies according to age, weight, the severity of pain and also the length of time that the medication has been used. Higher doses are needed if the medication has been taken on a regular basis. 5-10mg is the usual adult dose for acute pain. This is given every three to four hours if necessary. Narcotic addicted people may take many times this amount without ill effect as their bodies have adapted to the increased dose.
Common Side-Effects	Drowsiness, dizziness, nausea, vomiting, confusion and constipation are very common with methadone. Large doses can impair breathing. A lowering of blood pressure can occur.
Actions with other Drugs	Any medication which can cause sedation will add to the sedative side-effects of methadone. Sleep drugs, antihistamines, antidepressants, benzodiazepines and major tranquillisers will display this additive effect as will alcohol. Some antidepressants (MAO inhibitors) can cause a severe elevation in blood pressure.
Pregnancy, Breastfeeding	The babies of mothers taking methadone may suffer withdrawal symptoms after birth. It is not recommended during breastfeeding.
Special Features, Comments	Overdosage with this medication is possible. Drowsiness, difficulty in breathing and excessive sedation suggest overdosage and medical advice should be sought immediately. Methadone is a drug of addiction and can be habit forming. It should only be taken under strict medical supervision. Alcohol will increase the sedative effects of methadone. Driving or hazardous work should be undertaken with caution.

methyldopa

Trade Names	Aldomet, Dopamet, Hydromet, Metalpha
How Available	tablet, injection
Drug Group	Antihypertensive (blood pressure lowering) drug
Prescription	Yes
Major Uses	Methyldopa has been used for many years to reduce blood pressure. It can be used alone or in combination. The injectable form of the medication can be used to treat severe elevations in blood pressure. Methyldopa is often used late in pregnancy if blood pressure is elevated, as it provides good control with no evidence of harm to mother or baby.
How it Works	The action of methyldopa is not fully known. Its most prominent action is to act on blood pressure centres within the brain and lead to a decrease in the tone of arteries throughout the body.
Usual Dosage	250-500mg two to three times per day is the usual adult dose, though this may be substantially higher.
Common Side-Effects	Sedation, headache, depression, weakness and fever are all relatively common with methyldopa. Nausea, vomiting, a rash, sleep disturbances and nightmares are much less common. Methyldopa can cause an inflammation in the liver, a form of hepatitis. It can also give rise to a type of anaemia in which red cells are actually broken down by the body (haemolytic anaemia). Some antidepressants can adversely affect the blood pressure effects of methyldopa and lead to a serious rise in blood pressure.
Actions with other Drugs	Methyldopa may counteract the beneficial effects of levodopa in Parkinson's disease. Any drug which can cause drowsiness will add to the sedative effects of methyldopa.
Pregnancy, Breastfeeding	Methyldopa has been used in large numbers of women to control blood pressure during pregnancy, and it is one of the preferred medications to treat this problem. No adverse effects have been demonstrated on the mother or fetus. It does cross into breastmilk, so, even though no adverse effects on the new-born have been seen, it should be used only if necessary.
Special Features, Comments	Alcohol may increase the sedative effects of methyldopa. As with all blood pressure medications, the drug should not be stopped abruptly and alterations made only on medical advice.

metoclopramide

Trade Names	Gastrobid Continus, Gastromax, Maxolon, Migravess, Paramax (paracetamol), Parmid, Primeperan
How Available	tablet, liquid, injection
Drug Group	Anti-nausea drug
Prescription	Yes
Major Uses	The most common use for metoclopramide is to control nausea and vomiting due to most causes. It can also be used to help prevent reflux of acid to the oesophagus from the stomach.
How it Works	The exact way in which this medication acts is not clear, though it may increase the effect of the cholinergic nervous system on the gastro-intestinal tract. It assists emptying of the stomach contents to the duodenum. It increases the tone of muscle at the top of the stomach, helping to prevent stomach acid from returning to the oesophagus.
Usual Dosage	10mg three times per day is the usual adult dose. In children the dose depends on age and weight. Side-effects are more common in children, so accurate dosage with syrup is necessary.
Common Side-Effects	Drowsiness and tiredness are the most common side-effects. Other problems include constipation, diarrhoea, and headache. Occasionally movement disturbances such as in Parkinson's disease can occur. These usually disappear when the drug is stopped.
Actions with other Drugs	Any medication which can cause sedation will add to the sedative side-effects of metoclopramide. Sleep drugs, antihistamines, anti-depressants, strong analgesics and major tranquillisers will display this additive effect as will alcohol. Metoclopramide increases absorption of paracetamol, levodopa and tetracyclines and decreases digoxin absorption. Anti-cholinergic drugs will reduce the beneficial actions of metoclopramide as will narcotic analgesics. Any medication which may cause movement disorders may increase this adverse effect of metoclopramide.
Pregnancy, Breastfeeding	This medication has been used during pregnancy with no ill effects demonstrated. However, it is not recommended for use during pregnancy, especially the first trimester, as a safety precaution. It is not recommended for use with breastfeeding.
Special Features, Comments	Alcohol will increase the sedative effects of metoclopramide and may make nausea worse.

metoprolol

Trade Names	Arabralene, Betaloc, Co-Betaloc, Lopresor, Mepranix
How Available	tablet
Drug Group	Betablocker
Prescription	Yes
Major Uses	Metoprolol is most commonly used to treat raised blood pressure. It also may be used to treat angina (pain from an inadequate oxygen supply to the heart). It is sometimes also used after a heart attack to prevent further damage to the heart muscle. Some disturbances of heart rhythm may also be treated by metoprolol.
How it Works	The means by which metoprolol decreases blood pressure is not known. It decreases heart rate, and this is one of the reasons it is effective in angina, but this does not explain its ability to lower blood pressure. It has a direct effect on an area of the heart responsible for the rate the heart beats, controlling some rhythm disturbances.
Usual Dosage	50-100mg daily is the usual adult dose for blood pressure control.
Common Side-Effects	Tiredness and cold hands and feet are the most common side-effects. Sleep problems and increased dreams can occur.
Actions with other Drugs	Calcium antagonists may markedly reduce heart rate if given with betablockers. Cimetidine can increase the level of metoprolol in the blood. Other blood pressure tablets can cause low blood pressure if given at the same time. Drugs used for asthma can be less effective.
Pregnancy, Breastfeeding	Metoprolol has been used for the treatment of raised blood pressure in pregnant women without recognised adverse effects. It can lower the fetal heart rate, which may be important at the time of delivery. It is not recommended for use by nursing mothers.
Special Features, Comments	It can be dangerous to withdraw this drug suddenly as a rapid rise in blood pressure or increase in heart oxygen consumption may occur. An overdose of this medication can be serious and immediate medical attention should be sought. People with diseased arteries to the legs may have worsened symptoms if metoprolol is used. Unstable diabetics should avoid metoprolol as it may mask signs of a low blood glucose level. People with asthma or chronic bronchitis should avoid metoprolol. It may make their problems much worse. The drug may need to be stopped before a general anaesthetic.

metronidazole

Trade Names	Elyzol, Flagyl, Metrogel, Metrolyl, Metrotop, Zadstat
How Available	tablet, liquid, injection, ointment, suppository
Drug Group	Antibiotic (effective against protozoa)
Prescription	Yes
Major Uses	Metronidazole is an antibiotic used for a variety of infections, often caused by bacteria that thrive without oxygen (anaerobic bacteria) and caused by advanced single cell organisms, protozoa. These include infections such as brain abscesses, some pneumonias, bone infections, leg ulcers and infections after childbirth. Gardnerella, a common vaginal infection responds to metronidazole treatment. Giardiasis, a diarrhoeal infection, is treated with this drug. Topical cream is available to treat a facial skin disease called acne rosacea.
How it Works	Metronidazole prevents energy from being used within the cell of bacteria and protozoa, and also impairs the reproductive function of the cell.
Usual Dosage	The usual adult dose is 200-400mg three times daily. Treatment is for seven days, but can be considerably longer. Reduced doses are used for children, depending on age and weight.
Common Side-Effects	Nausea, vomiting, loss of appetite, abdominal pain and a metallic taste in the mouth are common side-effects with metronidazole. A furry tongue may be due to overgrowth with funguses. Occasionally, pins and needles in the hands and feet can occur with long-term use.
Actions with other Drugs	Alcohol should not be consumed during a course of treatment with metronidazole. This may produce severe adverse reactions including abdominal pain, sweating, nausea and vomiting. Metronidazole may increase the effect of anti-coagulants and phenytoin. Cimetidine may increase metronidazole in the body.
Pregnancy, Breastfeeding	This medication has not been proven safe in pregnancy, even though no definite problems have been demonstrated. It crosses into breastmilk, and is not recommended for nursing mothers.
Special Features, Comments	If metronidazole is continued for more than ten days then regular blood tests should be performed to make sure blood cells are being produced normally. It should not be given to people with blood disorders affecting white cells.

mianserin

Trade Names	Bolvidon, Norval
How Available	tablet
Drug Group	Tetracyclic antidepressant
Prescription	Yes
Major Uses	Mianserin is used for the treatment of depression, especially when the depression is accompanied by sleeping problems. It is most commonly used for elderly people and people with a history of heart disease.
How it Works	The exact mode of action of this group of drugs on the central nervous system is not known.
Usual Dosage	Most adults take 30-90mg per night as a single dose.
Common Side-Effects	When mianserin is started or the dose increased, drowsiness, tiredness and lethargy are common. Dry mouth, sweating, blurred vision, constipation and difficulty passing urine can occur, but are less common with this drug compared to other antidepressant tablets. Other side-effects have been reported in individual people.
Actions with other Drugs	All drugs, including alcohol, which have a sedative effect will have an additive effect on mianserin. Sleep drugs, antihistamines, other antidepressants, strong analgesics, benzodiazepines and major tranquillisers are the most common examples. Mianserin should not be used at the same time as another type of antidepressant (MAO inhibitors) as occasionally very serious side-effects may occur. Mianserin may alter the level of phenytoin in the blood.
Pregnancy, Breastfeeding	Safe use of this medication in pregnant women has not been established. Its use should be avoided if possible. Nursing mothers should also avoid the drug as it can pass into breast milk.
Special Features, Comments	Overdosage is possible with mianserin. Excessive tiredness, rapid pulse rate, low or high blood pressure should suggest possible overdosage. Immediate medical attention is imperative. Due to its sedative properties it is important not to drive or do dangerous work until the effect of the drug on the individual is established. Alcohol will increase sedation.

moclobemide

Trade Names	Manerix
How Available	tablet
Drug Group	Antidepressant (RIMA antidepressant)
Prescription	Yes
Major Uses	This drug is used for the treatment of a wide range of depressive illnesses.
How it Works	Moclobemide has similar net effects on the nervous system as another group of drugs (the monoamine oxidase inhibitors). However, unlike these drugs, moclobemide works on one particular type of this enzyme (MAO type A). The effect of this enzyme inhibition can also be reversed. This means that it has many fewer side-effects. The end result is similar, in changing the levels of neurotransmitters within the brain.
Usual Dosage	300mg per day is the recommended dose, however, up to 600mg may be used. It is not recommended for use in children.
Common Side-Effects	Insomnia, dizziness, nausea, dry mouth, constipation, diarrhoea, anxiety and restlessness are the most common side-effects. These are often transient. Other side-effects have been reported but are much less likely.
Actions with other Drugs	Unlike other MAO inhibitors it is generally safe to eat most foods, even foods rich in the amino acid tyramine. Eating such foods while using moclobemide does not cause a dramatic rise in blood pressure as it does with conventional MAO inhibitors. Also, it is generally safe to combine the use of moclobemide with other antidepressants. The medication may interact with cimetidine, so a lower dose of moclobemide may be necessary.
Pregnancy, Breastfeeding	Moclobemide has not been proven safe in pregnancy or breastfeeding, though no specific problems have been established. It can be used if thought necessary.
Special Features, Comments	Moclobemide has not been shown to have any particular interaction with alcohol. Even though a normal diet does not cause problems, it is still recommended that tyramine rich foods (cheese, red wine, Vegemite) be avoided. People with overactive thyroid conditions may require special care if using moclobemide. If overdose is suspected, urgent medical advice should be sought immediately.

morphine

Trade Names	Aspav, Cyclimorph, MST Continus, Oramorph, Sevredol, SRM Rhotard
How Available	tablet, liquid, injection, sustained release tablet
Drug Group	Narcotic analgesic
Prescription	Yes

Major Uses

Morphine is used for severe pain. It can be used for pain associated with severe injury, surgery, heart attack or abdominal pain. It is often used in advanced cancer to provide strong, effective pain relief.

How it Works

This medication is thought to act on specific receptors in the central nervous system leading to pain reduction.

Usual Dosage

The dose varies according to age, weight, the severity of pain and also the length of time that the medication has been used. Higher doses are needed if the medication has been taken on a regular basis. 5-25mg is the usual adult dose for acute pain. This is given every three to four hours if necessary.

Common Side-Effects

Drowsiness, dizziness, nausea, vomiting, confusion and constipation are very common with morphine. Large doses can impair breathing. Dry mouth, palpitations and an allergic rash can occur. A lowering of blood pressure is possible.

Actions with other Drugs

Any medication which can cause sedation will add to the sedative side-effects of morphine. Sleep drugs, antihistamines, antidepressants, benzodiazepines and major tranquillisers display this additive effect as will alcohol. Some antidepressants (MAO inhibitors) can cause a severe elevation in blood pressure.

Pregnancy, Breastfeeding

Morphine can cause a depression in respiration in the newborn. If it is used to control pain at the time of delivery a narcotic antagonist (e.g. naloxone) may need to be given to the baby. Its use is generally not recommended in pregnancy. The drug can pass into breastmilk, so mothers should avoid breastfeeding if they take the medication.

Special Features, Comments

Overdosage with this medication is possible. Drowsiness, difficulty in breathing and excessive sedation suggest overdosage and medical advice should be sought immediately. Morphine is a drug of addiction and can be habit forming if it is taken in large amounts for a prolonged period. It should only be taken under strict medical supervision. Alcohol will increase the sedative effects of morphine. Driving or hazardous work should be undertaken with caution.

naproxen

Trade Names	Napratec, Naprosyn, Narcan, Nycopren, Synflex
How Available	tablet, suppository, suspension, sustained release tablet
Drug Group	NSAID (non-steroidal anti-inflammatory drug)
Prescription	Yes, in most cases
Major Uses	Naproxen is a NSAID which is used in a variety of complaints including many types of arthritis and pain, and stiffness associated with inflammation of joints and soft tissues. Naproxen is often used to treat pain associated with menstrual periods, gout and migraine headaches.
How it Works	This drug prevents the action of substances (prostaglandins) which act on local tissues to produce pain and inflammation.
Usual Dosage	375-1250mg daily in divided doses, depending on nature of problem. Not usually recommended for children.
Common Side-Effects	All NSAIDs produce gastro-intestinal symptoms to some degree. These most commonly are nausea, vomiting, upper abdominal pain and heartburn. Occasionally an ulcer or bleeding from the stomach or duodenum may occur. Other possible side-effects include headache, dizziness, ringing in the ears and a rash. Suppositories may give rectal discomfort.
Actions with other Drugs	Use of this drug with aspirin or cortico-steroids may increase the chances of peptic ulcer and bleeding. The effect of blood pressure and fluid tablets (diuretics) may be reduced. It may interfere with anti-coagulant medications and can increase levels of lithium in the blood.
Pregnancy, Breastfeeding	Naproxen may cause fetal abnormalities early in pregnancy and can interfere with fetal blood circulation in the heart late in pregnancy. Thus, it is not recommended in pregnancy. It has been shown to pass into breast milk. Its use in breastfeeding should be discussed with your doctor.

continued over page...

naproxen continued

Special Features, Comments This medication should be given with caution in people with impaired liver or kidney function or in people with heart failure. Alcohol will increase the irritation of the stomach caused by naproxen. It should not be used in people with a history of peptic ulcer. The medication may interfere with clotting and this should be considered before surgery or dental work.

nicotine chewing gum

Trade Names	Niconil, Nicorette, Nicotinell
How Available	chewing gum
Drug Group	Anti-smoking treatment
Prescription	No, for low-strength gums. Yes for high strength.
Major Uses	Nicotine chewing gum is used alone or in addition to other forms of treatment to assist people give up smoking. In general, the treatment is more successful if used as part of a comprehensive behavioural smoking-cessation programme.
How it Works	Nicotine used over a long period can lead to a form of dependence on the drug. In using nicotine to help stop smoking, the aim is to divide the habit of smoking from the problem of drug dependence, so making quitting easier and more successful.
Usual Dosage	Nicotine chewing gum is used when the urge to smoke occurs. As the nicotine is absorbed rapidly from the mouth, blood nicotine levels will rise soon after a piece of active gum is chewed. The gum is usually chewed for a few seconds then left in the mouth between teeth and gum. This prevents excessive release of nicotine, which may cause side-effects. The number of pieces of gum used depends on the urge to smoke, and the number and strength of cigarettes previously smoked.
Common Side-Effects	Nausea, faintness and headache can occur if excessive nicotine enters the blood (too high a dose of gum or too frequent chewing). Some people complain of an unpleasant taste, excessive saliva and of the gum sticking to the teeth or dental work.
Actions with other Drugs	Other medications which lower blood pressure could possibly add to the effect of nicotine.
Pregnancy, Breastfeeding	The harmful effects of cigarette smoking are well documented. Some of these are due to the effects of nicotine. Therefore, nicotine should not be taken in pregnancy and women using nicotine gum should use effective contraception. Nicotine gum should not be used by breast-feeding mothers.
Special Features, Comments	Nicotine chewing gum should not be used after a heart attack or in people with angina (inadequate oxygen supply to areas of the heart muscle). It is possible that it may cause irritation to the stomach or irritate a peptic ulcer if swallowed.

nicotine patches

Trade Names	Nicotinell
How Available	skin patch
Drug Group	Anti-smoking treatment
Prescription	Yes

Major Uses

Nicotine patches can be used alone or with other types of treatment to assist people in giving up smoking. In general, the treatment is more successful if used as part of a comprehensive behavioural smoking cessation programme.

How it Works

Nicotine used over a long period can lead to a form of dependence on the drug. In using nicotine to help stop smoking, the aim is to divide the habit of smoking from the problem of drug dependence, so making quitting easier and more successful.

Usual Dosage

Skin patches come in various strengths. Smoking should be stopped at the time that treatment is commenced. At the start of treatment, the doctor decides on the strength of patch to be used. This depends on the number and strength of cigarettes smoked. Patches are left on for a period of 24 hours, and the site of the patch is changed daily. After treatment for approximately a month the patch strength is reduced and may be reduced again after a further few weeks. The maximum treatment course is 2-3 months.

Common Side-Effects

These may be due to therapy or actually giving up smoking. Common side-effects include headache, insomnia, tiredness, pain, sore throat, nausea, constipation, back pain, muscle pain, tiredness and menstrual pain. A rash may occur and skin irritation can occur under and around the patch site.

Actions with other Drugs

Nicotine has wide ranging effects on the body and smoking cessation or the use of patches may necessitate either an increase or decrease in the dose of other medications. Consult your doctor.

Pregnancy, Breastfeeding

The harmful effects of cigarette smoking are well documented. Some of these are due to the effects of nicotine. Therefore, nicotine should not be taken in pregnancy and women using nicotine patches should use effective contraception. Nicotine patches should not be used by breastfeeding mothers.

nicotine patches continued

Special Features, Comments
Smoking should cease before treatment is commenced. People with known ischaemic heart disease generally should avoid nicotine treatment. Nicotine treatment may impair the healing of peptic ulcers. Caution should be used in treating people with severe blood pressure problems and impaired liver function. Patches should be handled and disposed of with caution.

nicotinic acid

Trade Names	Cirflo, Hexopal, Nicotinic Acid, Proflo, TRI B3, Ronicol
How Available	tablet
Drug Group	Lipid lowering drug, vitamin
Prescription	No
Major Uses	Nicotinic acid has a number of uses. It is a naturally occurring vitamin. A severe deficiency of nicotinic acid leads to a condition known as pellagra, which can be treated successfully by nicotinic acid replacement. This medication is also used to lower blood cholesterol and triglycerides. As it dilates blood vessels, conditions in which there is poor circulation to the feet (e.g. chilblains and Raynaud's disease) can be treated using nicotinic acid.
How it Works	Nicotinic acid is essential to many human cells to ensure normal functioning. The way in which nicotinic acid causes a reduction in blood fats is not known. It does have a number of effects on lipid metabolism in the body, so it probably exerts its effects by a number of mechanisms. Nicotinic acid has a direct action on blood vessels, causing them to dilate.
Usual Dosage	Sometimes quite high doses 3-6g must be used to achieve adequate reductions in blood fats. Much lower doses (150-250mg) are used for the treatment of pellagra and to dilate blood vessels.
Common Side-Effects	One side-effect of nicotinic acid predominates. This is flushing and it can be severe enough to stop the drug. Other similar side-effects include dizziness, a fall in blood pressure, especially on standing, and headache. A rash, palpitations, nausea and vomiting can occur.
Actions with other Drugs	Other medications which lower blood pressure accentuate some of nicotinic acid's side-effects.
Pregnancy, Breastfeeding	Nicotinic acid is not recommended for use in pregnancy or breastfeeding (except as a vitamin supplement if there is a definite deficiency) although no specific problems have been demonstrated.
Special Features, Comments	Nicotinic acid should not be used in people with a history of peptic ulcers or recent heart attack. Blood tests will need to be performed for blood fats to assess response and to ensure that blood glucose and liver function are not adversely affected.

nifedipine

Trade Names	Adalat, Angiopine MR, Beta-adalat, Calcilat, Coracten, Nifensar XL, Tenif
How Available	tablet, capsule
Drug Group	Calcium channel blocker
Prescription	Yes
Major Uses	The most common use for nifedipine is for angina (pain in the chest due to insufficient oxygen supply to the heart muscle). In addition it can be used effectively for long term reduction of blood pressure. People with poor circulation to their limbs, for example Raynaud's disease, can be helped with this drug.
How it Works	Calcium channel blockers are thought to prevent the flow of calcium in the walls of smooth muscle cells which line small arteries. This decreases blood pressure, increases flow through the arteries and prevents spasm of the walls of arteries (which occurs in the heart in some attacks of angina). Nifedipine may actually reduce the amount of oxygen consumed by the heart muscle.
Usual Dosage	30-60mg daily is the usual adult dose for angina prevention and the treatment of high blood pressure. In addition 5-10mg can be taken to treat an actual episode of angina. It is not generally used in children.
Common Side-Effects	Ankle swelling, dizziness, headache, excessively low blood pressure when standing. Nausea and light-headedness are common. Most of these reflect the way nifedipine works. They usually occur at the start of treatment and disappear or decrease with time.
Actions with other Drugs	Nifedipine increases the effects of drugs which lower blood pressure. Beta-blocker medications can act at a similar place in the heart conduction system and possibly lead to a serious slowing of heart rate. Heart conduction problems can also occur if nifedipine is used with digoxin or amiodarone. Cimetidine increases the effects of nifedipine.
Pregnancy, Breastfeeding	Birth defects are theoretically possible if this drug is used in pregnancy, so it is generally not used. It is not recommended for nursing mothers, though no definite problems have been established.
Special Features, Comments	Nifedipine should be used cautiously in people with severe heart failure. Alcohol may accentuate the blood pressure lowering properties of the drug and may cause more side-effects.

nitrazepam

Trade Names	Mogadon, Somnite
How Available	tablet
Drug Group	Benzodiazepine
Prescription	Yes
Major Uses	Nitrazepam is used for the short-term treatment of insomnia. It usually induces a sleep which lasts for 6-8 hours.
How it Works	The exact action of this drug and of other drugs in the benzodiazepine group is not known. It works on the central nervous system.
Usual Dosage	2.5-10mg at night before retiring.
Common Side-Effects	Drowsiness, dizziness, confusion and headache are all common side-effects with nitrazepam use. Occasionally, agitation and over-activity may result, even with normal doses. Side-effects are more frequent in elderly people.
Actions with other Drugs	Any medication which can cause sedation will add to the sedative side-effects of nitrazepam. Sleep drugs, antihistamines, antidepressants, strong analgesics and major tranquillisers will display this additive effect as will alcohol.
Pregnancy, Breastfeeding	This medication is not recommended in pregnancy or breastfeeding. An infant can develop withdrawal symptoms if the drug is used up to delivery, and it can pass into breast milk.
Special Features, Comments	As with other benzodiazepines, there is a potential for dependence with long term use of the medication. Also overdosage can occur. Excessive sleepiness and the inability to rouse a person who has access to nitrazepam should lead to the suspicion of overdosage. Immediate medical attention is necessary. Alcohol should be avoided with nitrazepam treatment. Driving and dangerous work situations should be performed with caution.

nitrofurantoin

Trade Names	Furadantin, Macrobid, Macrodantin
How Available	tablet, liquid
Drug Group	Antibiotic
Prescription	Yes
Major Uses	Nitrofurantoin is an antibiotic used for bacterial infections of the urinary tract e.g. bladder and kidney infections.
How it Works	This medication acts on a number of bacterial enzyme systems to halt the growth of the organism, though in the urine it is in higher concentrations and it actually kills bacteria.
Usual Dosage	50-100mg four times per day is the usual adult dose. Maximum dose is 400mg per day. This dose is reduced in children according to age and weight.
Common Side-Effects	Nausea is quite common with nitrofurantoin, though this may be decreased by taking the medication with something to eat. Abdominal pain and diarrhoea can occur as can inflammation of the liver. Rarely, damage to nerves may cause numbness in the feet. If tingling occurs, especially if the person treated has other medical problems, the drug should be stopped at once. Headache, dizziness and a rash may occur as can a fever. Inflammation in the lung tissue, anaemia and alteration in white cells in the blood can occur, but are rare.
Actions with other Drugs	Probenecid will increase the level of nitrofurantoin in the blood. Nitrofurantoin decreases the effect of norfloxacin.
Pregnancy, Breastfeeding	If given late in pregnancy or in breastfeeding, the drug may be transmitted to the baby, and perhaps cause a type of anaemia. For this reason it is not generally used in late pregnancy, or while breastfeeding.
Special Features, Comments	Nitrofurantoin is not usually give for long periods, due to its potential side-effects.

nizatidine

Trade Names	Axid
How Available	tablet
Drug Group	Anti-ulcer drug
Prescription	Yes
Major Uses	Nizatidine is used for the treatment of ulcers in the stomach and duodenum. Following healing of an ulcer, the drug is usually continued for a period, in order to prevent recurrence. Nizatidine can also be used to decrease inflammation caused by stomach acid in the oesophagus (reflux oesophagitis).
How it Works	Nizatidine is a type of drug known as a H2 (histamine 2) receptor antagonist. This means that it blocks the action of histamine on the cells of the stomach which are responsible for acid production. The net result is a dramatic decrease in acid production. Accordingly, there is a decrease in the acid irritation to the oesophagus, stomach and duodenum, allowing healing of an ulcer.
Usual Dosage	300mg once daily in the evening or 150mg twice per day is the usual adult dose. The maintenance dose is 150mg in the evening. This can be continued for up to 12 months. This medication is not often prescribed for children.
Common Side-Effects	This drug is generally well tolerated, and side-effects are rare. These include sweating, a rash and sleepiness. Other side-effects are much less likely.
Actions with other Drugs	Unlike cimetidine (another drug of this group), nizatidine does not have any substantial interactions with other medications.
Pregnancy, Breastfeeding	Although no special problems have been demonstrated with nizatidine and breastfeeding, it should only be used if necessary.
Special Features, Comments	Alcohol and cigarettes can delay ulcer healing, so they are best avoided while using nizatidine. Dosage should be reduce in people with severe kidney problems.

norethisterone

Trade Names	BiNovum (with ethinyloestradiol), Brevinor (with ethinyloestradiol), Menzol, Micronor, Noriday, Noristerat, Primolut-N, Utovlan
How Available	tablet
Drug Group	Oral contraceptive
Prescription	Yes
Major Uses	Norethisterone is similar to a naturally occurring female sex hormone (progesterone). It is used in many types of oral contraceptive pills, either alone (the progesterone only or 'mini-pill') or in combination with oestrogen. It is also used in combination with oestrogen after the menopause and sometimes to treat irregular menstrual bleeding. Occasionally, it is used to treat inoperable breast cancer.
How it Works	If used alone as a contraceptive, norethisterone most likely acts by altering the nature of mucus around the cervix, preventing sperm from fertilising the ovum. In combination with oestrogen it prevents release of hormones which stimulate the ovary. As a result no ova are released. Its ability to reduce hormone release from the brain is the basis for its use in breast cancer.
Usual Dosage	0.35mg per day is the usual dose of norethisterone in progesterone only pills. It is important that the dose be taken at the same time every day to achieve effective contraception. Slightly higher doses 0.5-1mg are used in combined pills. Much higher doses 5-20mg are used to treat menstrual disorders.
Common Side-Effects	Change in menstrual periods and irregular menstrual bleeding are common side-effects if the medication is used alone. Weight gain and swollen ankles may also occur. Other potential side-effects are possible if used with oestrogen. (See ethinyloestradiol.)
Actions with other Drugs	Many antibiotics can interfere with norethisterone and combination contraceptive pills leading to irregular bleeding and, sometimes, contraceptive failure. It is important to let your doctor know if you are taking any other medications when norethisterone is prescribed.
Pregnancy, Breastfeeding	Norethisterone is used in women who are breastfeeding and need contraception. Small amounts of norethisterone do pass into the breastmilk, but have not been shown to cause problems.
Special Features, Comments	If used for long periods at high doses, blood tests may be necessary to check liver function.

norfloxacin

Trade Names	Utinor
How Available	tablet
Drug Group	Antibiotic (quinolone antibiotic)
Prescription	Yes

Major Uses

Norfloxacin is largely used in the treatment of urinary tract infections. It is effective against most bacteria that cause these. In addition, it may be effective in treating traveller's diarrhoea and occasionally other infections of the bowel.

How it Works

This medication exerts its effect by interfering with the reproduction of bacterial cells. It does this in a number of ways, killing the bacteria.

Usual Dosage

One tablet (400mg) twice per day before meals for seven to ten days is the usual adult dose for urinary tract infections, though a course for three days is adequate for most infections. A five day treatment course is recommended for traveller's diarrhoea. Norfloxacin may interfere with joint formation, so it is not used in children.

Common Side-Effects

Nausea, dizziness and headache are the most common side-effects of norfloxacin, though it is generally well tolerated. Fatigue, rash and abdominal pain may occur. Other side-effects are rare. Occasionally, an impairment of liver function may occur.

Actions with other Drugs

Probenecid will increase the level of norfloxacin in the blood. Antacids may decrease the absorption of norfloxacin. Nitrofurantoin may decrease the antibiotic action of norfloxacin.

Pregnancy, Breastfeeding

Quinolone antibiotics as a group are thought to interfere with joint formation in young animals. For this reason, it is advised that pregnant women and nursing mothers avoid using norfloxacin, though no specific problems have been established.

Special Features, Comments

A reduced dose of norfloxacin should be used in people with reduced kidney function, and sometimes elderly people.

nortriptyline

Trade Names	Allegron, Motipress, Motival
How Available	tablets
Drug Group	Tricyclic antidepressant
Prescription	Yes
Major Uses	This medication is used in the treatment of depression. The antidepressant effects start after two to three weeks of treatment.
How it Works	The exact mode of action of this group of drugs on the central nervous system is not known.
Usual Dosage	10-75mg daily is the usual adult dose. The medication is not usually prescribed in children.
Common Side-Effects	When nortriptyline treatment is commenced, drowsiness, dry mouth, blurred vision, constipation and difficulty passing urine may occur. These effects often diminish with time. Other side-effects can occur on an individual basis.
Actions with other Drugs	Sleep drugs, antihistamines, strong analgesics, benzodiazepines and major tranquillisers will add to the sedative effects of nortriptyline as will alcohol. Nortriptyline and other tricyclic antidepressants should not be used at the same time as another type of antidepressant (MAO inhibitors) as occasionally very serious side-effects may occur. Nortriptyline may reduce the effect of some blood pressure reducing drugs. Smoking and barbiturates can reduce the antidepressant effect of this drug.
Pregnancy, Breastfeeding	Safe use of this medication in pregnant women has not been established. Its use should be avoided if possible. Nursing mothers should also avoid the drug as it can pass into breast milk.
Special Features, Comments	All tricyclic antidepressants including nortriptyline can have serious consequences if an overdose is taken as eventually they will have a profound effect on the heart. Dizziness, blurred vision, dry mouth, agitation, convulsions and lack of arousal should give rise to suspicion of overdosage. Immediate medical attention is imperative. Due to its sedative properties it is important not to drive or to perform hazardous work until the effect of the drug on the individual is established. Alcohol will increase sedation. Nortriptyline is not generally given to people with a history of heart disease.

nystatin

Trade Names	Nystan in combination: Dermovate-NN, Flagyl Campak, Gregoderm, Nystadermal, Nystaform, Terra-Cortril, Nystatin, Timodine, Tinaderm-M, Tri-Adcortyl, Tricicatrin, Trimovate
How Available	syrup, pessary, powder, tablet, cream, lotion
Drug Group	Antifungal antibiotic
Prescription	Yes
Major Uses	Nystatin has a wide variety of uses against many types of fungal infections. It generally works against the fungi responsible for athlete's foot, tinea and ringworm as well as many others. Pessaries are used for vaginal infections and syrups for mouth infections. When taken by mouth, it can treat some fungal infections in the gastro-intestinal tract.
How it Works	Nystatin acts on the fungus cell wall and membranes changing the environment within fungus cells preventing their normal functioning.
Usual Dosage	Topical: apply to the affected area up to three times daily. Treatment should continue for several days following cessation of symptoms to prevent recurrence. Oral: 2-4 million units per day is used for most fungal gastro-intestinal infections.
Common Side-Effects	These are uncommon. Occasionally, a local stinging may occur, or redness and itchiness to the skin. Local allergic reactions are possible. Occasionally, diarrhoea, nausea, vomiting and abdominal bloating may occur with the oral medications.
Actions with other Drugs	Nil of note.
Pregnancy, Breastfeeding	There is no evidence that nystatin adversely affects the fetus. The vaginal cream and pessaries are often used to treat fungal infections in pregnant women and are generally considered safe. It is safe to use while breastfeeding.
Special Features, Comments	There is no specific problem in taking the oral medications with alcohol.

omeprazole

Trade Names	Losec
How Available	tablet
Drug Group	Anti-ulcer drug
Prescription	Yes
Major Uses	Omeprazole is used in the treatment of peptic ulcers. It is effective for stomach and duodenal ulcers and may be of benefit in reducing inflammation caused by acid in the esophagus. (It is of particular use in a condition known as the Zollinger-Ellison syndrome, a very rare cause of peptic ulcers.)
How it Works	This medication works by preventing the enzyme responsible for stomach acid production from functioning effectively. This prevents hydrogen ions from being pumped from the cell into the stomach, decreasing acid production, reducing inflammation and allowing ulcer healing.
Usual Dosage	20mg every day is the usual adult dose for the treatment of ulcers. This is usually continued for 4-8 weeks. At present, omeprazole is not recommended for long term use nor is it used in children.
Common Side-Effects	Nausea, diarrhoea, headache, abdominal pain, flatulence and dyspepsia are the most common side-effects seen, though the medication is generally well tolerated. A skin rash has occurred occasionally.
Actions with other Drugs	Omeprazole causes an increase in the blood levels of diazepam and phenytoin. It also increases the anticoagulant activity of warfarin.
Pregnancy, Breastfeeding	Omeprazole is not recommended for use in pregnancy or breastfeeding, although no specific problems have been demonstrated.
Special Features, Comments	Omeprazole should be used with caution in people with liver disease.

ondansetron

Trade Names	Zofran
How Available	tablet, intravenous solution
Drug Group	Anti-nausea drug
Prescription	Yes
Major Uses	This drug is used essentially for the treatment of nausea and vomiting caused by the chemotherapy and radiotherapy of various types of cancer.
How it Works	Ondansetron is a very potent blocker of the $5HT_3$ receptor in the body. The exact mechanism by which this prevents nausea and vomiting is unknown, but it is presumed that many of the causes of nausea and vomiting following chemotherapy are due to the release of 5HT (5-hydroxytryptamine).
Usual Dosage	This varies depending on the type of chemotherapy. Initially a dose is given intravenously and followed by an oral dose of 8mg three times per day for 5 days. In children the dose is approximately half the adult dose.
Common Side-Effects	Headache, a sensation of flushing, constipation, altered taste are common side-effects. Other problems are much less likely.
Actions with other Drugs	Ondansetron has been shown to be compatible with a wide range of drugs used in the treatment of cancer. It is usually administered at the same time as the anti-cancer drugs.
Pregnancy, Breastfeeding	It is not recommended that ondansetron be used in pregnant or breastfeeding women, unless the potential benefits outweigh possible problems. It is unlikely that it would be used in either.
Special Features, Comments	Ondansetron is a major advance in the treatment of nausea and vomiting in the treatment of cancer.

oxazepam

Trade Names	Oxazepam
How Available	tablet
Drug Group	Benzodiazepine
Prescription	Yes
Major Uses	Oxazepam has a variety of uses including treatment of sleep problems, anxiety, agitation and tension. It can be used to treat the agitation of alcohol withdrawal.
How it Works	The exact action of this drug and of other drugs in the benzodiazepine group is not known. It works on the central nervous system.
Usual Dosage	15-30mg per dose. One dose at night (insomnia), or three to four doses through the day (agitation) is the usual dosage range.
Common Side-Effects	Mild drowsiness over the first few days of treatment is the most common side-effect. This usually diminishes considerably after the first few days. Dizziness, headache, nausea and confusion occur with higher doses. Other side-effects are less frequent. Side-effects are more frequent in elderly people.
Actions with other Drugs	Any medication which can cause sedation will add to the sedative side-effects of nitrazepam. Sleep drugs, antihistamines, antidepressants, strong analgesics and major tranquillisers will display this additive effect as will alcohol.
Pregnancy, Breastfeeding	This medication is not recommended in pregnancy or breastfeeding. An infant can develop withdrawal symptoms if the drug is used up to delivery, and it can pass into breast milk.
Special Features, Comments	As with other benzodiazepines, there is a potential for dependence with long term use of the medication. Overdosage can occur. Excessive sleepiness and the inability to arouse a person who has access to nitrazepam should lead to the suspicion of overdosage. Immediate medical attention is advised. Alcohol should be avoided with oxazepam treatment. Driving and hazardous work situations should be performed with caution.

oxprenolol

Trade Names	Slow-Trasicor, Trasicor, Trasidrex
How Available	tablet
Drug Group	Betablocker
Prescription	Yes
Major Uses	Oxprenolol is most commonly used to treat raised blood pressure. It also may be used to treat angina (pain from inadequate oxygen supply to the heart). Some disturbances of heart rhythm may also be treated by oxprenolol. Some effects of an over-active thyroid can be reduced by oxprenolol.
How it Works	The means by which oxprenolol decreases blood pressure is not known. It decreases the heart rate, and this is one of the reasons it is effective in angina, but does not explain its ability to lower blood pressure. It has a direct effect on an area of the heart responsible for the rate of heart beat, controlling some rhythm disturbances.
Usual Dosage	80-160mg twice daily is the average adult dosage.
Common Side-Effects	Tiredness, cold hands and feet, sleep disturbances and nightmares are the most common side-effects. Dizziness and depression can also occur.
Actions with other Drugs	Calcium antagonists may reduce heart rate if given with betablockers. Indomethacin may decrease oxprenolol's blood pressure reduction capacity. Drugs used for asthma can be less effective.
Pregnancy, Breastfeeding	Oxprenolol is not recommended in pregnancy unless benefits outweigh potential risks. It can lower the fetal heart rate, which may be important at the time of delivery. It is not suggested for use by nursing mothers.
Special Features, Comments	It can be dangerous to withdraw this drug suddenly as a rapid rise in blood pressure or increase in heart oxygen consumption may occur. People with diseased arteries to the legs may have worse symptoms if oxprenolol is used. Unstable diabetics should avoid oxprenolol as it may mask signs of a low blood glucose level. People with asthma or chronic bronchitis should avoid oxprenolol. It may make their problems considerably worse. The drug may need to be stopped before a general anaesthetic is given. An overdose of this medication can be serious and immediate medical attention should be sought.

paracetamol

Trade Names	Paracetamol is used alone or in combination in many over the counter and prescription medications such as Alvedon, Calpol, Cosalgesic, Distalgesic, Fortagesic, Kapake, Lobak, Medised, Midrid, Migraleve, Paldesic, Pameton, Panadol, Paramax, Propain, Remedeine, Salzone, Solpadol, Sudafed-co, Syndol, Tylex, Uniflu
How Available	tablet, capsule, liquid, suppository
Drug Group	Analgesic, anti-pyretic
Prescription	No
Major Uses	Paracetamol is used extensively in cases of mild to moderate pain and to reduce fever. It does not treat the cause of the pain or fever.
How it Works	The exact way in which paracetamol eases is not well known.
Usual Dosage	Adult doses are usually 500mg-1g. The dosage in children varies with age and weight. Most preparations have doses for children clearly indicated on the label. In both adults and children, the dose may be repeated every four hours.
Common Side-Effects	Paracetamol is generally very well tolerated. It does not cause an inflammation to the stomach or interfere with blood clotting, so it is safe to use in people with peptic ulcers. Occasionally a rash or nausea may occur.
Actions with other Drugs	In high doses, paracetamol may interfere with oral anticoagulant drugs. Cholestyramine (Questran) may prevent paracetamol from being absorbed.
Pregnancy, Breastfeeding	Paracetamol has been used extensively during pregnancy and in breastfeeding. It has not been shown to be a problem for the mother, fetus or newborn infant. It is regarded as safe to use.
Special Features, Comments	Overdosage can cause severe damage to the liver. Many times the normal dose must be taken if this is to occur. There may be no symptoms of overdose until irreparable damage to the liver has occurred (usually 2-3 days later). However, if overdose is treated early, liver damage can be prevented. Alcohol may increase the inflammation of the liver in this situation. If paracetamol does not lead to resolution of pain or fever promptly, medical advice should be sought to establish the cause of the problem.

penicillamine

Trade Names	Distamine, Pendramine
How Available	tablet
Drug Group	Anti-inflammatory drug
Prescription	Yes
Major Uses	The most common use for penicillamine is to treat rheumatoid arthritis (a long term inflammation of joints and other tissues). Penicillamine can also be used to bind with heavy metals and remove them from the body. It removes copper, lead and mercury from the body. An abnormal accumulation of copper (Wilson's disease) is treated by penicillamine. Cystinuria, a rare disease, will also respond to treatment with this drug.
How it Works	The way penicillamine acts in rheumatoid arthritis is not known. It may interfere with antibody components of the immune reaction. In other diseases, penicillamine binds with the offending substance and makes it more soluble, allowing it to pass into the urine.
Usual Dosage	A dose of 125mg per day is the usual starting dose, though this is increased to a level of 750mg to 1g as maintenance dose for rheumatoid arthritis. For Wilson's disease a daily dose of 1-2g is needed. Metal poisoning may require a lower dose. The dose in children depends on weight, age and the disease treated.
Common Side-Effects	A rash, nausea, vomiting and loss of the sensation of taste are the commonest side-effects. Other potential problems include a number of changes to red and white cells in the blood, liver inflammation and kidney disease. Degeneration of vision can occur. Iron supplements may be needed for women on penicillamine treatment.
Actions with other Drugs	The action of isoniazid is enhanced by penicillamine, the action of digoxin decreased. Antacids reduce the absorption of penicillamine.
Pregnancy, Breastfeeding	Penicillamine may cause birth defects. It should not be given during pregnancy. Use of this medication during breastfeeding is not recommended.
Special Features, Comments	Blood and urine tests are monitored at regular intervals. Eyes should be examined every six months. Pyridoxine (vitamin B6) and iron supplements may be useful for people on long term treatment. supervision. Alcohol will increase the sedative effects of pentazocine. Driving or hazardous work should be undertaken with caution.

pentazocine

Trade Names	Fortagesic, Fortral
How Available	tablet, injection
Drug Group	Narcotic analgesic
Prescription	Yes
Major Uses	Pentazocine is used for moderate to severe pain. It can be used for pain associated with severe injury, before or after surgery or in childbirth. It is often used in cancer and chronic pain to provide strong, effective pain relief.
How it Works	This medication is thought to act on specific receptors in the central nervous system to lead to a reduction in pain.
Usual Dosage	The dose varies according to age, weight, the severity of pain and also the length of time that the medication has been used. Higher doses are needed if the medication has been taken on a regular basis. 25-100mg is the usual adult dose for acute pain. This is given every four hours if necessary. Lower doses are used in children.
Common Side-Effects	Drowsiness, nausea, vomiting, dizziness and confusion can occur. Impairment of breathing can occur with large doses. An increase in blood pressure is possible.
Actions with other Drugs	Sleep drugs, antihistamines, antidepressants, benzodiazepines, major tranquillisers and alcohol will add to the sedative effect of pentazocine. Some antidepressants (MAO inhibitors) can cause a severe elevation in blood pressure. The absorption of phenytoin may be impaired by pentazocine.
Pregnancy, Breastfeeding	Pentazocine can cause depression in respiration in the newborn. If it is used to control pain at the time of delivery a narcotic antagonist (e.g. naloxone) may need to be given to the baby. Its use is generally not recommended in pregnancy. The drug can pass into breast milk, so mothers should avoid breastfeeding if they must take the medication.
Special Features, Comments	Overdosage causes drowsiness, difficulty in breathing and excessive sedation. Medical advice should be sought immediately. Pentazocine is a drug of addiction and can be habit forming if taken for a prolonged period. It should only be taken under strict medical supervision. Alcohol will increase the sedative effects of pentazocine. Driving or hazardous work should be undertaken with caution.

perindopril

Trade Names	Coversyl
How Available	tablet
Drug Group	ACE inhibitor (angiotensin converting enzyme inhibitor)
Prescription	Yes
Major Uses	This medication is most commonly used for the long-term treatment of raised blood pressure.
How it Works	This drug is converted into active form by the liver after absorption in the gut. Perindopril works mainly by preventing the action of angiotensin converting enzyme in transforming angiotensin I to angiotensin II. Angiotensin II is a very active substance, so stopping its formation generally leads to a reduction in blood pressure.
Usual Dosage	2-8mg per day as a single dose. This medication has not been proven safe for children, and is not recommended for their use.
Common Side-Effects	Headache, weakness, dizziness, nausea, abdominal pain and cough are the commonest side-effects and may require discontinuing the medication. There are numerous other effects, but they are much less common. ACE inhibitors often cause a taste disturbance which subsides after 1-3 months of treatment.
Actions with other Drugs	Excessive lowering of blood pressure may occur in people taking other blood pressure medication, and especially fluid tablets. As ACE inhibitors prevent the loss of potassium, drugs which add or spare potassium are generally not given at the same time. Perindopril may cause a rise in serum lithium levels.
Pregnancy, Breastfeeding	Perindopril and other ACE inhibitors are not recommended for use in pregnancy as they may cause birth defects. It is not advised for use by nursing mothers.
Special Features, Comments	ACE inhibitors should be used with caution in people with impaired kidney function and in people with narrowing of their heart valves. Older patients may be more susceptible to the medication. Even though the drug is activated by the liver, impaired liver function does not appear to affect the metabolism of the drug. Tests on blood chemistry may be necessary from time to time.

pethidine

Trade Names   Pamergan P100, Pethidine

How Available   tablet, injection

Drug Group   Narcotic analgesic

Prescription   Yes

Major Uses   Pethidine is used for severe pain. It can be used before or after surgery, for pain associated with severe injury and to relieve pain during childbirth. It is not generally used for chronic pain or cancer pain.

How it Works   This medication is thought to act on specific receptors in the central nervous system leading to a reduction in pain.

Usual Dosage   The dose varies according to age, weight and severity of the pain. 50-100mg is the usual adult dose for acute pain. This is given every three to four hours if necessary.

Common Side-Effects Nausea, vomiting, dizziness, drowsiness, confusion and constipation are the most common side-effects of pethidine. Large doses can impair breathing. Hallucinations and a lowering of blood pressure can occur.

Actions with other Drugs Any medication which can cause sedation will add to the sedative side-effects of pethidine. Sleep drugs, antihistamines, antidepressants, benzodiazepines and major tranquillisers will display this additive effect as will alcohol. Some antidepressants (MAO inhibitors) can cause a severe elevation in blood pressure.

Pregnancy Breastfeeding Pethidine can cause depression in respiration in the newborn. As it is commonly used to control pain at the time of delivery a narcotic antagonist (e.g. naloxone) may need to be given to the baby. The drug can pass into breastmilk, but as the drug is not continued for long periods after delivery it is not usually of concern.

Special Features, Comments Overdosage with pethidine causes drowsiness, difficulty in breathing and excessive sedation. Medical advice should be sought immediately. Pethidine is a drug of addiction and can be habit forming if it is taken in large amounts for a prolonged period. It should only be taken under strict medical supervision. Alcohol will increase the sedative effects of pethidine. Driving or hazardous work should be undertaken with caution.

phenelzine

Trade Names	Nardil
How Available	tablet
Drug Group	Antidepressant (MAO inhibitor)
Prescription	Yes
Major Uses	Phenelzine is a member of a group of drugs known as mono-amine oxidase inhibitors (MAO inhibitor). These medications are used to treat severe depression and are very effective in improving mood, increasing activity and appetite. They are usually used when another medication with fewer potential side-effects has failed.
How it Works	The action of MAO inhibitors is widespread. They stop the break down of a number of important nerve transmission substances, by blocking the action of the enzyme mono-amine oxidase. They may also act in other ways as well.
Usual Dosage	45mg is the usual starting dose for adults. This may be increased to as high as 90mg to achieve the full antidepressant effect. This may take up to four weeks after treatment is begun. After the desired effect is achieved the dose is slowly lowered as much as possible. This medication is not recommended for children.
Common Side-Effects	In most situations phenelzine is well tolerated. Most common side-effects include dizziness, dry mouth, light-headedness, an excessive fall in blood pressure when standing, constipation and weakness. A rash, nausea and vomiting and a headache may occur. Inflammation of the liver is rare. Euphoria and agitation can occur.
Actions with other Drugs	The major problem with the use of MAO inhibitors is that they interact with many other medications and even some foods e.g. cheeses, Vegemite and red wine. The most serious adverse reaction is a sudden and potentially dangerous increase in blood pressure. Many medications, even cough remedies and non-prescription drugs, may cause this reaction. It is imperative that medical advice be sought before any additional medication is taken. Other antidepressant medications should not be given during or for a three week period after stopping phenelzine treatment as other potentially serious problems may occur.

phenelzine continued

Pregnancy, Breastfeeding
Phenelzine is not recommended for use in pregnant or breastfeeding women, though no specific problems have been established. As some drugs used in delivery may interact with phenelzine, it is usually stopped four weeks before delivery.

Special Features, Comments
Phenelzine should not be used in people with epilepsy or liver disease. Before the medication is started baseline blood tests are usually taken. Phenelzine should not be given to people over sixty, people with raised blood pressure or reduced arterial flow to the heart or brain. Phenelzine should be stopped two weeks before any planned general anaesthetic. Red wine can cause a serious reaction with phenelzine. Other alcohol should be avoided. Driving and dangerous work should be undertaken with caution. Overdose with phenelzine is possible, with sweating and fever being common symptoms. If suspected, immediate medical advice should be sought.

phenindione

Trade Names	Dindevan
How Available	tablet
Drug Group	Oral anticoagulant
Prescription	Yes

Major Uses

Phenindione is used to prevent and treat blood clots within blood vessels. It can be used to treat clots in the veins of the leg, and to prevent recurrence of clots in the lung vessels (pulmonary emboli). It is sometimes used as an alternative to warfarin, if this medication causes an allergic reaction.

How it Works

This medication works by antagonising the action of vitamin K in the liver. This leads to a decrease in the formation of some clotting factors, hence the action of the body's major natural clotting mechanism is restricted and clots much less likely to form. Often phenindione therapy is begun in hospital and may follow on from treatment with an intravenous drug, heparin.

Usual Dosage

When phenindione is started, the full anti-clotting effect does not take place for two to three days. Often a higher than normal daily dose is given for the first day or two of treatment. Once stable, doses of 25-100mg twice daily is the usual adult dose range. Strict monitoring of the clotting capacity of the blood is necessary. This is done by measuring the prothrombin ratio (an easily performed blood test). This is normally kept in a therapeutic range of 2-4 for people on phenindione treatment. Phenindione dosage varies greatly with each individual and also with time.

Common Side-Effects

The most common and potentially serious side-effect of phenindione therapy is abnormal bleeding. Black, tarry bowel motions are often the first indicator of a bleed from the gastro-intestinal tract. This can occur even if the medication is in the therapeutic range. Any unusual symptoms should be reported to a doctor. Other side-effects include fever, nausea, diarrhoea and allergic rash. Rarely severe allergic reactions can occur.

phenindione continued

Actions with other Drugs

Many drugs are known to increase or decrease the anticoagulant effect of phenindione, even non-prescription drugs. It is vital that medical advice be sought before any other drug is taken. If another medication is introduced, a change to the phenindione dose will often be necessary. Aspirin may prolong the effect of phenindione and may increase the chances of bleeding.

Pregnancy, Breastfeeding

Oral anticoagulant may cause fetal abnormalities and fetal death and should not be used in pregnancy. If an oral anticoagulant is needed in breastfeeding, then warfarin is preferred to phenindione. This is because phenindione is secreted in breastmilk even at therapeutic doses, unlike warfarin.

Special Features, Comments

Regular blood tests are vital to the long term successful use of phenindione. Phenindione needs to be stopped or other anticoagulant medications used before surgery or dental work, to avoid excessive bleeding. Alcohol may alter the dose of phenindione needed. Any illness e.g. infections, heart disease, recent surgery or liver disease will either increase or decrease the effect of phenindione. Phenindione should not be used in people with bleeding disorders e.g. haemophilia, or in people with ulcers or bleeding areas in the gastro-intestinal or urinary tract. It should not be used in people with severe liver or kidney disease.

phenoxymethylpenicillin (penicillin V)

Trade Names	Penicillin V
How Available	tablet, liquid, injection
Drug Group	Antibiotic (penicillin)
Prescription	Yes

Major Uses This form of penicillin is used for a large number of infections. However, because many infections are resistant to penicillin or do not respond, it is not used for as many problems as other penicillin based antibiotics. Phenoxymethylpenicillin is used for some skin infections and some bacterial infections of the throat. It can be used for dental and gum infections. It is given to people with damaged heart valves to prevent bacterial infections in the valves.

How it Works This medication is thought to interfere with the manufacture of bacterial cell walls, eventually leading to the destruction of the bacteria.

Usual Dosage The adult dose is usually 250-500mg four times daily. It is important that the medication be taken one hour before or two hours after meals as a full stomach interferes with absorption. Dosage in children depends on weight, age and the infection being treated.

Common Side-Effects A rash is the commonest side-effect of phenoxymethylpenicillin. (More severe allergic reactions are much less common. A severe rash or difficulty in breathing requires immediate medical assessment.) Nausea and vomiting as well as diarrhoea are also common side-effects. Other side-effects can occur with higher doses.

Actions with other Drugs Antacids will reduce the absorption of phenoxymethylpenicillin if taken at the same time. Probenecid increases the blood level of this penicillin and is actually sometimes given to achieve this result. Phenoxymethylpenicillin may reduce the effectiveness of the oral contraceptive pill.

Pregnancy, Breastfeeding This medication has been used extensively during pregnancy and no special problems have been demonstrated. It is generally considered safe to use in pregnancy and breastfeeding.

Special Features, Comments Overgrowth of fungus in the mouth, gastro-intestinal tract and vagina may occur especially if used for prolonged periods.

phentermine

Trade Names	Duromine, Ionamin
How Available	tablet
Drug Group	Drug for weight reduction
Prescription	Yes
Major Uses	Phentermine is used as an adjunct to diet to achieve weight loss.
How it Works	This drug acts on the central nervous system to reduce the feeling of hunger thereby reducing food intake. Reduced calorie intake will eventually lead to a decrease in weight.
Usual Dosage	15-40mg daily.
Common Side-Effects	Insomnia, restlessness, agitation, tremor, palpitations and elevation in blood pressure are possible problems as are dry mouth, nausea and vomiting.
Actions with other Drugs	Phentermine can interact with some antidepressant medications. It may decrease the dose of insulin necessary for some diabetics. Phentermine may counteract the effect of blood pressure lowering drugs. It should not be given with other weight control tablets. It can make the stimulant effects of coffee and nicotine more pronounced.
Pregnancy, Breastfeeding	This medication is not usually recommended for use in pregnancy or breastfeeding.
Special Features, Comments	Treatment is usually for three continuous months. Treatment will only be effective if accompanied by a decrease in dietary intake. Long-term weight reduction will only occur if patterns of food use change. It should not be used in people with raised eye pressure (glaucoma) or in people with a history of agitation or drug abuse. Driving and hazardous work should be undertaken with caution.

phenytoin

Trade Names	Epanutin, Pentran
How Available	tablet, syrup
Drug Group	Anticonvulsant (drug used in epilepsy)
Prescription	Yes

Major Uses
This medication is effective in the treatment of a wide variety of seizures including grand mal and temporal lobe seizures. Phenytoin is used to prevent seizures e.g. after operations on the brain, following head injuries or where other brain damage has occurred. It can also be used in the treatment of migraine and occasionally for heart rhythm disturbances.

How it Works
Phenytoin acts on the motor cortex in the brain to stop spreading of electrical stimuli which cause seizures.

Usual Dosage
150-600mg daily is the normal adult dose range depending on the type of problem treated and the response. Children's doses also depend on age and weight.

Common Side-Effects
A relatively common side-effect of phenytoin, which may stop treatment, is overgrowth of gum tissue. Gums affected may impair the health of teeth and also bleed easily. Dizziness, unsteadiness, sedation, confusion and nausea are also common. Rarely, blood cell production may be interfered with, a potential worry as the drug is intended for long-term use.

Actions with other Drugs
Many medications can alter the level of phenytoin in the blood. Anticoagulants, barbiturates and phenylbutazone are some of these. Ethosuximide and carbamazepine, both used for epilepsy, can also interfere with the phenytoin level. Some antidepressants may cause unusual body movements if used with phenytoin. Phenytoin may decrease the effectiveness of the oral contraceptive pill.

phenytoin continued

Pregnancy,
Breastfeeding

Women who use anticonvulsant drugs during pregnancy do have an increased chance of birth defects. The chance is about three times normal. Phenytoin use in pregnancy can cause growth and mental retardation, and some specific deformities of the face in the fetus. In many cases, there is no alternative but to use phenytoin. The potential problems to mother and baby of uncontrolled fitting during pregnancy outweigh the possibility of having an abnormal child. The drug is passed into breastmilk and safety in breastfed infants has not been proven.

Special Features,
Comments

Due to the sedative effects of the drug, driving and dangerous work should be undertaken with caution. Blood tests at regular intervals are usually taken to assess the level of phenytoin in the blood. Alcohol can increase the sedative effect of the drug.

pilocarpine

Trade Names	Isopto Carpine, Minims pilocarpine nitrate, Ocusert Pilo, Sno Pilo
How Available	eye drops, eye inserts
Drug Group	Drug for glaucoma
Prescription	Yes
Major Uses	This medication is most commonly used to lower eye pressure in some types of glaucoma. It may also be used to counteract the effects of other medications used to dilate the pupil for eye examinations.
How it Works	Pilocarpine acts by stimulating that segment of the nervous system (the parasympathetic nervous system) which leads to a stimulation of the muscle in the iris responsible for pupil constriction.
Usual Dosage	Eye drops are generally used every six to eight hours. Slow release inserts are changed every seven days. The medication is not generally used in children.
Common Side-Effects	Blurred vision, headaches, irritation to the eyes are all common side-effects with this medication. Allergic reactions may occur.
Actions with other Drugs	None have been reported.
Pregnancy, Breastfeeding	No problems have been found in pregnant women using these eye drops. They are used if necessary. The drug will pass into breastmilk and it is not generally used in this situation.
Special Features, Comments	The eye may become used to the effects of the drug and another medication may need to be substituted if it becomes less effective.

pindolol

Trade Names	Viskaldix, Visken
How Available	tablet
Drug Group	Betablocker
Prescription	Yes
Major Uses	Pindolol is most commonly used to treat raised blood pressure. It also may be used to treat angina (pain from an inadequate oxygen supply to the heart). Some disturbances of heart rhythm may also be treated by pindolol.
How it Works	The means by which pindolol decreases blood pressure is not known. It decreases the heart rate, and this is one of the reasons it is effective in angina, but this does not explain its ability to lower blood pressure. It has a direct effect on an area of the heart responsible for the rate at which the heart beats, controlling some rhythm disturbances.
Usual Dosage	15mg per day is the most frequently prescribed adult dose.
Common Side-Effects	Dizziness, tiredness, weakness, sleep disturbances, nausea and vomiting are the most common side-effects. There are many other, but much less frequent, side-effects.
Actions with other Drugs	Pindolol will add to the effect of other blood pressure lowering drugs. Calcium antagonists may markedly reduce heart rate if given with betablockers.
Pregnancy, Breastfeeding	Pindolol is not recommended for use in pregnancy unless benefits outweigh potential risks. It can lower fetal heart rate, which may be important at the time of delivery. It is not suggested for use by nursing mothers.
Special Features, Comments	It can be dangerous to withdraw this drug suddenly as a rapid rise in blood pressure or increase in heart oxygen consumption may occur. People with diseased arteries to the legs may have worse symptoms if pindolol is used. Unstable diabetic patients should avoid pindolol as it may mask signs of a low blood glucose level. People with asthma or chronic bronchitis should avoid pindolol. It may make their problems considerably worse. The drug may need to be stopped before a general anaesthetic is given. An overdose of this medication can be serious and immediate medical attention should be sought.

piroxicam

Trade Names	Feldene
How Available	capsule, dispersible tablet
Drug Group	NSAID (non-steroidal anti-inflammatory drug)
Prescription	Yes
Major Uses	Piroxicam is a NSAID which is used in a variety of complaints including many types of arthritis and stiffness associated with inflammation of joints and soft tissues. It can be used to treat gout.
How it Works	This drug prevents the action of substances (prostaglandins) which act on local tissues to produce pain and inflammation.
Usual Dosage	10-20mg daily as a single dose. Not recommended for children.
Common Side-Effects	All NSAIDs produce gastro-intestinal symptoms to some degree. These most commonly are nausea, vomiting and upper abdominal pain. Piroxicam can also cause flatulence. Dizziness, a rash and breathlessness can occur. It is rare, but possible for piroxicam to produce an ulcer in the stomach or duodenum and this may bleed. (For this reason any person with a history of ulcer disease should avoid piroxicam and NSAIDs generally.)
Actions with other Drugs	Use of this drug with aspirin or cortico-steroids may increase chances of peptic ulcer and bleeding. It should not be used in people with peptic ulcers. This medication may raise the level of digoxin or lithium in the blood. The effect of blood pressure and fluid tablets (diuretics) may be reduced. It may interfere with the effect of anti-coagulant medications. Piroxicam may increase the action of methotrexate (a drug used for cancer and rheumatoid arthritis) with severe effects on the bone marrow.
Pregnancy, Breastfeeding	Piroxicam may delay the onset and progress of labour and may also interfere with the baby's blood circulation in the heart late in pregnancy. It is not recommended in pregnancy and has been shown to cross over to the infant in breast milk, so use in breast-feeding should be discussed with your doctor.
Special Features, Comments	This medication should be given with caution in people with impaired liver, kidney or heart function. Alcohol increases irritation of the stomach. Piroxicam may interfere with clotting. This should be considered before surgery or dental work.

pizotifen

Trade Names	Sanomigran
How Available	tablet
Drug Group	Anti-migraine drug
Prescription	Yes
Major Uses	Pizotifen is used to prevent migraine headaches. It is also used to prevent other headaches which are caused by blood vessel dilation. These include atypical migraine and headaches known as cluster headaches. The medication can only be used to prevent headaches, it is of no use in treating the headache itself.
How it Works	The exact way in which pizotifen prevents migraine headaches is not known. It does interfere with serotonin, which may be responsible for the dilation of blood vessels around the brain, the cause of migraine. Pizotifen does have other actions, being a mild anti-depressant and antihistamine.
Usual Dosage	One to three tablets per day is the usual dose in adults. A lower dose is used if the medication is required for children.
Common Side-Effects	Weight gain is a common occurrence with the long term use of pizotifen (it increases appetite). Dizziness and drowsiness can occur. Dry mouth, headache, constipation and a rash are all possible, but uncommon side-effects.
Actions with other Drugs	Any medication which can cause sedation will add to the sedative side-effects of pizotifen. Sleep drugs, benzodiazepines, antihistamines, antidepressants, strong analgesics and major tranquillisers will display this additive effect as will alcohol. Some antidepressants (MAO inhibitors) can cause a dangerous rise in blood pressure. Medications which have anticholinergic effects can add to the severity of the dry mouth and constipation caused by pizotifen.
Pregnancy, Breastfeeding	Though no specific problems have been established with the use of pizotifen in either pregnancy or breastfeeding, its use is not recommended.
Special Features, Comments	Alcohol will increase the sedative side-effects of pizotifen and should be avoided while the drug is being used. Driving and dangerous work should be undertaken with extreme caution.

pravastatin

Trade Names	Lipstat
How Available	tablet
Drug Group	Lipid lowering drug
Prescription	Yes
Major Uses	Pravastatin is used for the treatment of most types of raised cholesterol. It is effectively only as long as it is taken, and does not eliminate the cause of the elevated blood cholesterol. It is important to adhere to a low cholesterol diet while the medication is taken.
How it Works	This drug acts by inactivating an enzyme (HMG CoA reductase) which is responsible for one of the first steps in the formation of cholesterol in the liver. (Most of the body's cholesterol is made within the body, rather than being taken in as food.) As a result the amount of cholesterol produced by the body is reduced.
Usual Dosage	The medication is commenced after a trial of a cholesterol lowering diet. The usual dose is 10 to 20mg per day at bedtime. This medication is not recommended for children.
Common Side-Effects	Nausea, vomiting, flatulence, constipation, diarrhoea, abdominal pain, heartburn, fatigue, a rash, headache and muscle pain are the commonest side-effects. Many other problems have been reported, but are much less likely.
Actions with other Drugs	Taking gemfibrozil (another lipid lowering drug) may impair removal of pravastatin from blood. The two drugs are generally not given together.
Pregnancy, Breastfeeding	It is thought that this group of drugs could cause birth defects, so pravastatin should not be used in pregnancy. It is not recommended for use during breastfeeding.
Special Features, Comments	Muscle pain and inflammation may occur with the use of HMG CoA reductase inhibitors. Adverse effects on liver function are sometimes noted with this drug. It is important to check liver function tests before, and at regular intervals during therapy.

prazosin

Trade Names	Hypovase
How Available	tablet
Drug Group	Antihypertensive (blood pressure lowering) drug
Prescription	Yes
Major Uses	Prazosin is most often used to lower raised blood pressure. It may also be used to treat heart failure. People with arterial spasm to the blood vessels of the hands and feet (Raynaud's disease) may benefit from prazosin treatment as may men with prostate obstruction.
How it Works	Prazosin acts by blocking effects of sympathetic nerve transmission and by dilating the small arterial blood vessels of the body. This leads to a fall in blood pressure and, as a result, an increase in the efficiency of the pumping action of the heart.
Usual Dosage	As the first dose of this medication may cause a marked fall in blood pressure, a very small dose, 0.5mg, is given first. This is increased slowly up to a maximum of 20mg until the appropriate response is achieved. Prazosin is usually given two to three times per day. It is not given to children less than twelve years of age.
Common Side-Effects	Dizziness and faintness are the most common, especially when treatment is started. Palpitations, lack of energy, nausea, headache, stuffy nose, blurred vision and dry mouth can occur.
Actions with other Drugs	Any other medication which lowers blood pressure will enhance the blood pressure lowering activity of prazosin.
Pregnancy, Breastfeeding	Prazosin is not recommended for use in pregnancy, although it has been used to lower blood pressure when other medications have proved inadequate. Some prazosin appears in breast milk, so its use is not recommended for nursing mothers.
Special Features, Comments	Prazosin should be given with caution to elderly people, as the drop in blood pressure when standing (postural hypotension) can be pronounced and sudden loss of consciousness may occur. It is possible that angina (lack of oxygen to the heart muscle) may be made worse by prazosin. Patients with liver disease may require a lower dose. Alcohol may increase the postural hypotension of prazosin. The dose should not be altered except under medical supervision, as a substantial rise in blood pressure may occur. If treatment is interrupted consult your doctor.

prednisolone/prednisone

Trade Names	Deltacortril, Deltastab, Minims prednisolone, Predenema, Predfoam, Pred Forte, Predsol, Scheriproct
How Available	tablet, injection, suppository, ointment, eye drops, ear drops
Drug Group	Corticosteroid
Prescription	Yes
Major Uses	This medication has a wide variety of uses. Mainly it is an anti-inflammatory agent used for local inflammatory problems to the skin, ears and eyes. The injectable form may be used to decrease inflammation. Prednisolone can be used to treat severe asthma. Tablets can be taken orally if the body is deficient in corticosteroids, or if extra corticosteroids are necessary. Prednisolone has many other uses in inflammatory and blood disorders.
How it Works	Prednisolone is very similar to a hormone produced by the body and it replaces this natural substance when taken by mouth. The exact way that it reduces inflammation in the skin and other sites is unknown, though one important effect is preventing cells which cause inflammation from arriving at the inflamed tissue.
Usual Dosage	This varies widely according to the nature and severity of the condition being treated. Topical preparations are used two to three times per day.
Common Side-Effects	All corticosteroids can produce a similar range of side-effects. If taken orally these include indigestion, nausea, weight gain, acne, weakness and thin bones. Peptic ulcer may occur. These side-effects usually occur with long-term treatment. Mood changes are possible with higher doses. Topical preparations can lead to thinning of the skin if used continuously. A rash may also occur. Use of topical medications does not lead to similar oral side-effects of the drug as little is absorbed with topical application.
Actions with other Drugs	Barbiturates, phenytoin, the oral contraceptive pill and rifampicin may decrease the available amount of prednisolone in the blood. Prednisolone may impair the control of diabetes with insulin or oral tablets and also interfere with blood pressure control. Vaccination should be delayed until treatment with prednisolone is ceased. Prednisolone may increase the side-effects of digoxin.

prednisolone/prednisone continued

Pregnancy, Breastfeeding
Corticosteroids, given orally, may increase the risk of birth defects, and decrease the baby's weight. At the end of pregnancy however, if a premature birth is anticipated, a short course of corticosteroids may help to prevent respiratory distress in the premature infant. Otherwise, prednisolone is used only if absolutely necessary. It is generally avoided in breastfeeding, as it passes into breastmilk.

Special Features, Comments
Blood tests at regular intervals may be necessary. Checks should be made from time to time to ensure that glaucoma (raised eye pressure) and diabetes are not present. Alcohol may increase the chance of peptic ulcer if taken with oral prednisolone.

probenecid

Trade Names	Benemid
How Available	tablet
Drug Group	Drug for gout
Prescription	Yes
Major Uses	Probenecid is used for the treatment of gout. It prevents attacks, but is not effective once an attack of gout has started. This medication is also used to increase the blood level and length of action of some antibiotics, especially penicillin antibiotics.
How it Works	This medication decreases the blood level of uric acid (the cause of gout attacks). It does this by preventing the reabsorption of uric acid in the kidney, once it has been filtered from the blood. Probenecid also interferes with the excretion of certain medications by the kidneys. A higher blood level is achieved with a lower dose of the other medication.
Usual Dosage	Usual adult dose is 0.5-1g twice daily. Children's dosage depends on age and weight. (Not given in children under two years.)
Common Side-Effects	Headache, nausea, vomiting, allergic skin rashes and dizziness are possible side-effects. In people who have gout, the attack may be made worse if probenecid is being used when the attack occurs. Occasionally, probenecid can cause uric acid kidney stones.
Actions with other Drugs	Many medications are affected by the use of probenecid. In some, blood levels are increased (many anti-inflammatory drugs, some antibiotics and oral blood glucose lowering drugs). Others are decreased. (These include aspirin, some diuretic tablets and alcohol.) Care should be taken if methotrexate (an anti-cancer and rheumatoid arthritis drug) is used at the same time, as it may cause serious problems even in normal doses.
Pregnancy, Breastfeeding	Probenecid should be used in pregnancy only if potential benefits outweigh risks. No specific problems in pregnancy have been established, however. The drug does pass into breastmilk and its use is not recommended unless absolutely necessary.
Special Features, Comments	People with blood diseases, or peptic ulcers should avoid probenecid. Blood tests are taken at regular intervals if the medication is used for long periods.

probucol

Trade Names	Lurselle
How Available	tablet
Drug Group	Lipid lowering drug
Prescription	Yes
Major Uses	Probucol is prescribed on its own or with other medications to lower blood cholesterol levels. It should be used in conjunction with a low cholesterol diet for maximum effect. Probucol treatment is usually reserved for people who have not responded to other types of treatment. Maximum effect of probucol occurs after one to three months.
How it Works	The exact way in which this medication works is not known. It has a number of effects on cholesterol metabolism, and decreases some of the lipids in the blood, either by preventing their formation or increasing their destruction.
Usual Dosage	Probucol is not recommended for children. The usual adult dose is 1g daily.
Common Side-Effects	Diarrhoea, nausea and vomiting, dizziness and abdominal pain are the most common side-effects of this medication. Numbness and palpitations can occur. Many other side-effects can occur, but are rare.
Actions with other Drugs	No significant interactions with other medications have been reported. Probucol adds to the cholesterol lowering effects of other drugs.
Pregnancy, Breastfeeding	Probucol's use is not recommended either in pregnancy or breastfeeding, though no specific problems have been shown. Further, because probucol lasts for a prolonged period of time in the body, women are advised to cease the medication some six months before becoming pregnant, and to use contraceptives while on the drug.
Special Features, Comments	Blood tests are taken at regular intervals to assess the medication's effect in lowering cholesterol.

procainamide

Trade Names	Procainamide Durules, Pronestyl
How Available	tablet, sustained release tablet, injection
Drug Group	Heart rhythm drug
Prescription	Yes
Major Uses	Procainamide is used to prevent and treat rapid heart rhythms and also to decrease the numbers of extra beats that the heart may produce.
How it Works	This medication works on a number of places within the heart to affect the transmission of heart impulses. The end result is a decrease in the heart's response to electrical stimuli and the control of rhythm.
Usual Dosage	2-4g per day is the usual dose. This should be given every 4-6 hours unless the sustained release tablet is used (increasing the interval between doses to every twelve hours).
Common Side-Effects	Nausea, vomiting and loss of appetite are the most common side-effects of procainamide treatment. Dizziness and weakness and allergic reactions may occur. Occasionally, symptoms similar to SLE (systemic lupus erythematosus) can occur, leading to joint pains, fever, a rash and some abnormal blood tests suggestive of the disease. This will usually disappear when the drug is stopped.
Actions with other Drugs	Although procainamide does not usually decrease blood pressure, this should be monitored if blood pressure lowering agents are used at the same time. Cimetidine can increase the level of procainamide in the blood.
Pregnancy, Breastfeeding	Although no specific problems have been demonstrated with procainamide in pregnancy or breastfeeding, the medication is generally not used unless absolutely necessary.
Special Features, Comments	Tests for SLE and blood cell function are usually performed if procainamide is used for long periods. People with severe liver or kidney disease may require lower doses of procainamide. The drug can make some rhythm disturbances worse and care must be taken, especially when the medication is started or the dose altered, to ensure that this does not occur.

prochlorperazine

Trade Names	Buccastem, Stemetil
How Available	tablet, injection, suppository
Drug Group	Anti-nausea drug
Prescription	Yes
Major Uses	Prochlorperazine is used to treat nausea and vomiting from motion sickness and other illnesses. It is also useful in Merniere's disease (a disease of the inner ear). In higher doses prochlorperazine can be used as a tranquillising medication.
How it Works	This medication acts on many centres within the brain. Many of its effects are due to the antagonism of a nerve transmitter substance (dopamine).
Usual Dosage	The adult dose for the treatment of nausea and vomiting is 5-10mg orally or 25mg by suppository. Prochlorperazine is not used in children less than two years of age as side-effects are more common.
Common Side-Effects	Drowsiness, dry mouth and constipation are common side-effects. Of some concern is the ability of this drug to cause involuntary movements and symptoms similar to those seen in Parkinson's disease. Movement disorders are potentially more serious in children. A rash and tremor are possible adverse reactions.
Actions with other Drugs	Any medication which can cause sedation will add to the sedative side-effects of prochlorperazine. Sleep drugs, antihistamines, antidepressants, strong analgesics and major tranquillisers will display this additive effect as will alcohol. The effect of some medications used for Parkinson's disease are reduced. Anti-cholinergic drugs will accentuate some of the side-effects of prochlorperazine.
Pregnancy, Breastfeeding	Prochlorperazine is not recommended for use in pregnancy or breastfeeding. It is known that it may cause movement problems after birth, if used by the mother during labour.
Special Features, Comments	Longer term use of prochloperazine may lead to a persistent movement disorder. Alcohol will increase the sedative effects of this drug. Driving or dangerous work should be undertaken with caution. People with severe liver disease may have delayed metabolism of prochlorperazine.

promethazine

Trade Names	Avomine, Medised suspension (with paracetamol), Pamergan P100 (with pethidine), Phenergan, Sominex
How Available	tablet, liquid, injection
Drug Group	Antihistamine
Prescription	No
Major Uses	Promethazine is a long acting antihistamine used to ease symptoms of respiratory infections and also in many allergic conditions e.g. hay fever and allergic eye conditions. Promethazine can ease the itch of many allergic skin rashes. It can also be used to stop the nausea of motion sickness or cancer. In children, it is sometimes used as a sedative if illness makes sleep difficult.
How it Works	Antihistamines prevent histamine from reacting with cells and causing local inflammation. (Histamine is a naturally occurring substance present in some white blood cells [mast cells]). The sedative and anti-nausea effects of promethazine occur as this drug crosses from the blood into the brain.
Usual Dosage	25mg three times daily is the adult dose for allergic problems. The dose in children depends on age, weight and the problem treated.
Common Side-Effects	Sedation, dizziness, tiredness, nausea and dry mouth are the most common side-effects. Blurred vision and paradoxical restlessness may occur, though this and other side-effects are much less common.
Actions with other Drugs	Any medication which can cause sedation will add to the sedative side-effects of promethazine. Sleep drugs, antihistamines, antidepressants, benzodiazepines, strong analgesics and major tranquillisers will display this additive effect as does alcohol.
Pregnancy, Breastfeeding	If used late in pregnancy, promethazine can cause prolonged movement disorders in newborn children. Though no specific problems have been demonstrated at other times in pregnancy or lactation, promethazine is not recommended in either.
Special Features, Comments	An overdose of promethazine can be a serious problem, because of the marked sedative effects of the drug. Inability to rouse a person, convulsions or difficulty in breathing should raise the suspicion of overdose. Immediate medical assistance should be sought. Driving and hazardous work should be undertaken with extreme caution. Alcohol should be avoided while promethazine is taken.

propranolol

Trade Names	Bedranol, Berkolol, Beta-Prograne, Inderal, Inderetic, Inderex
How Available	tablet
Drug Group	Betablocker
Prescription	Yes

Major Uses

Propranolol is most commonly used to reduce blood pressure. It has many other uses including treatment of over-active thyroid, some types of tremor, the prevention of migraine headaches and some heart rhythm problems. Propranolol may also be used to treat angina (pain from an inadequate oxygen supply to the heart). It is sometimes also used after a heart attack to prevent further damage to the heart muscle.

How it Works

The means by which propranolol decreases blood pressure is not known. It decreases the heart rate, and this is one of the reasons it is effective in angina, but this does not explain its ability to lower blood pressure. It has a direct effect on an area of the heart responsible for the rate at which the heart beats, controlling some rhythm disturbances.

Usual Dosage

The dose varies depending on the type and severity of the problems being treated. For raised blood pressure the dose is 40-160mg twice daily, occasionally higher.

Common Side-Effects

Tiredness, cold hands and feet, nausea, sleep disturbances and vivid dreams are the most common side-effects. Other side-effects can occur, but are infrequent.

Actions with other Drugs

Calcium antagonists may markedly reduce heart rate if given with betablockers. Cimetidine increases the level of propranolol in the blood. Other blood pressure tablets can cause low blood pressure if given at the same time. Drugs used for asthma can be less effective.

Pregnancy, Breastfeeding

Propranolol has been used for the treatment of raised blood pressure in pregnant women without recognised adverse effects. It is not recommended unless benefits outweigh potential risks. It can lower the fetal heart rate, which may be important at the time of delivery. It is not suggested for use by nursing mothers.

continued over page...

propranolol continued

**Special Features,
Comments**

It can be dangerous to withdraw this drug suddenly as a rapid rise in blood pressure or increase in heart oxygen consumption may occur. People with diseased arteries to the legs may have worsened symptoms if propranolol is used. Unstable diabetics should avoid propranolol as it may mask signs of a low blood glucose level. People with asthma or chronic bronchitis should avoid propranolol. It may make their problems much worse. The drug may need to be stopped before a general anaesthetic is given. An overdose of this medication can be serious and immediate medical attention should be sought.

propylthiouracil

Trade Names	Not yet available in the UK
How Available	tablet
Drug Group	Antithyroid drug
Prescription	No
Major Uses	Propylthiouracil (PTU) can be used in the most common form of an over-active thyroid gland, Graves' disease. Long term treatment of this condition is possible with PTU, but it is more commonly used when the initial diagnosis of Graves' disease is made, before thyroid surgery or radioactive iodine treatment is given or during pregnancy.
How it Works	PTU blocks the conversion of thyroxine (the hormone produced by the thyroid gland) into the active form of the hormone (tri-iodothyronine). This effectively decreases the action of the thyroid gland on the body.
Usual Dosage	200-400mg daily in three to four doses is the usual initial dose for adults, though the maintenance dose varies considerably. Dosage in children depends on weight and age.
Common Side-Effects	PTU is generally well tolerated. An itch or rash and dizziness are the most common side-effects. Jaundice is possible. Of the less common side-effects, the most worrying is the potential depression of blood cell formation. It may also interfere with the blood's ability to clot and lead to bleeding. A sore throat and jaundice are possible. Liver function and blood clotting tests may be affected.
Actions with other Drugs	Anticoagulant drugs may interact with PTU to cause bleeding problems.
Pregnancy, Breastfeeding	PTU can be used in pregnancy, but there is a risk that it may interfere with the thyroid function of the fetus, or cause goitre. If it is necessary to use PTU, then the lowest possible dose should be given and the baby watched closely for evidence of impaired thyroid function. PTU is excreted in breastmilk and should not be used while breastfeeding.
Special Features, Comments	Tests for thyroid function and blood cell function are taken regularly on people using PTU.

pyrantel

Trade Names	Combantrin
How Available	tablet, suspension, granules
Drug Group	Anti-helminth (anti-worm) drug
Prescription	No
Major Uses	Pyrantel is a single dose treatment for most worm infestations of the gastro-intestinal tract. These include roundworm, threadworm and hookworm.
How it Works	This medication works by preventing nerve transmission within the nervous systems of worms, effectively paralysing them, resulting in eradication of the infestation.
Usual Dosage	Dosage in adults and children is adjusted on the basis of weight. The usual dose is 10mg of pyrantel base per kilogram of body weight as a single dose. If one family member is affected by threadworm, then generally the whole family is treated.
Common Side-Effects	Nausea, vomiting, lack of appetite, diarrhoea, dizziness, headache and a rash have all been reported, but are not common. Occasionally mild abnormalities in liver function may occur.
Actions with other Drugs	Nil known.
Pregnancy, Breastfeeding	There is no evidence of fetal abnormalities with the use of pyrantel. It can be used if necessary, though it should be avoided till after pregnancy, if possible.
Special Features, Comments	Pyrantel is not recommended for use in people with liver disease.

quinapril

Trade Names	Accupro, Accuretic
How Available	tablet
Drug Group	ACE inhibitor (Angiotensin converting enzyme inhibitor)
Prescription	Yes
Major Uses	This medication is most commonly used for the long-term treatment of raised blood pressure.
How it Works	Quinapril works mainly by preventing the action of angiotensin converting enzyme in transforming angiotensin I to angiotensin II. Angiotensin II is a very active substance, so stopping its formation generally leads to a reduction in blood pressure.
Usual Dosage	5-10mg once per day before meals is the usual dose, but up to 40mg may be necessary. This medication has not been proven safe for children, and is not recommended for their use.
Common Side-Effects	Headache, dizziness, fatigue, coughing, nausea, vomiting and abdominal pain are the most common side-effects and may require cessation of therapy. Other side-effects are less likely. ACE inhibitors often cause a taste disturbance which subsides after 1-3 months of treatment.
Actions with other Drugs	Excessive lowering of blood pressure may occur in people taking other blood pressure medication, and especially fluid tablets. As ACE inhibitors prevent the loss of potassium, drugs which add or spare potassium are generally not given at the same time. Quinapril may cause a rise in serum lithium levels. Indomethacin may decrease the efficacy of quinapril. Quinapril may impair the absorption of tetracyclines.
Pregnancy, Breastfeeding	Quinapril and other ACE inhibitors are not recommended for use in pregnancy as they may cause birth defects. It is not advised for use by nursing mothers.
Special Features, Comments	Quinapril absorption is affected by meals, so it should be taken before food. ACE inhibitors should be used with caution in people with impaired kidney function and in people with narrowing of their heart valves. Older patients may be more susceptible to the medication. Tests on blood chemistry may be necessary from time to time.

quinidine

Trade Names	Kinidin Durules
How Available	sustained release tablet
Drug Group	Heart rhythm drug
Prescription	Yes
Major Uses	Quinidine is used in the treatment of some heart rhythm disturbances. It is often used to attempt to slow the heart rate by converting an abnormal rhythm to normal.
How it Works	This medication interferes with the flow of sodium into the heart muscle cell and the flow of potassium out of the heart muscle cell during contraction. This has a number of effects on the various stages of transmission of the electrical impulse through the heart.
Usual Dosage	600mg to 1.8g is the usual adult dose. If the medication is not sustained release it must be given three to four times per day as it only acts for a short time in the body. The medication is not generally prescribed for children.
Common Side-Effects	Diarrhoea, nausea, vomiting, dizziness and abdominal pain are common side-effects with quinidine treatment. Sometimes unintended heart rhythm disturbances may occur, as may blurred vision and ringing in the ears. If used for a long time some of the symptoms and abnormal blood tests of a condition known as SLE (systemic lupus erythematosus) may occur. An allergic rash is possible.
Actions with other Drugs	Quinidine may increase the level of digoxin in the blood. As they may be used together, it is often necessary to reduce the dose of digoxin. People on digoxin treatment as well as quinidine may be more susceptible to some heart rhythm problems. Also, quinidine may increase the effect of oral anticoagulant drugs.
Pregnancy, Breastfeeding	Quinidine should not be used in either pregnancy or breastfeeding. It may cause an increased risk of fetal death and deformities. The drug can pass into breastmilk.
Special Features, Comments	Blood tests may be necessary with long term use of quinidine to check on blood levels of the drug, and for other possible problems. Overdose with quinidine can occur. This may be suspected if fits or breathing problems occur. Heart rhythm may be affected. If suspected, immediate medical attention is essential.

quinine

Trade Names	Not yet available in the UK
How Available	tablet
Drug Group	Drug for malaria and muscle cramps
Prescription	No
Major Uses	Quinine is most commonly used to relieve nocturnal muscle cramps. It has been a treatment for malaria for many years, and is still used for treating severe infections, however quinine is not generally used for malaria prevention because of its toxic effects.
How it Works	This medication has a number of actions on muscle. It diminishes the action of a nerve transmitter (acetylcholine) at the nerve-muscle junction and also increases the minimum time between responses that the muscle can make to stimuli, thus making spasm less likely and relieving cramps. Quinine acts on one phase of the malaria parasite cycle, causing death to some forms of the parasite only.
Usual Dosage	300mg at night is the usual adult dose for cramps. The dose to treat malaria is considerably higher. For malaria treatment, age and weight determine the dose in children.
Common Side-Effects	There is a low ratio between toxic and therapeutic levels of quinine in the blood. Symptoms of excess quinine are common. These include nausea, headache and ringing in the ears. Other side-effects include itching, loss of hearing and blood disorders (such as a dramatic reduction in platelet numbers), but these are rare.
Actions with other Drugs	Quinine increases the level of digoxin in the blood. The effect of anticoagulants may be increased.
Pregnancy, Breastfeeding	Quinine should not be used in either pregnancy or breastfeeding. It may cause fetal death and deformities. The drug can pass into breastmilk and is not recommended for use in breastfeeding.
Special Features, Comments	Overdose with quinine can occur. This is usually heralded by hearing and breathing problems. Heart rhythm may be affected. If suspected, immediate medical attention should be sought. In the doses needed to treat nocturnal cramps, no long term problems are expected. Quinine should not be used in people with impaired eye or ear function.

ramipril

Trade Names	Tritace
How Available	capsule
Drug Group	ACE inhibitor (Angiotensin converting enzyme inhibitor)
Prescription	Yes
Major Uses	This medication is most commonly used for the long-term treatment of raised blood pressure.
How it Works	Ramipril is absorbed in the gut and converted in the liver to its active form. It works mainly by preventing the action of angiotensin converting enzyme in transforming angiotensin I to angiotensin II. Angiotensin II is a very active substance, so stopping its formation generally leads to a reduction in blood pressure.
Usual Dosage	2.5-10mg per day in a single dose. This medication has not been proven safe for children, and is not recommended for their use.
Common Side-Effects	Nausea, dizziness, headache and cough may occur as can vomiting, abdominal pain and a rash. These side-effects may require cessation of the drug. Other problems are less likely. ACE inhibitors often cause a taste disturbance which subsides after 1-3 months of treatment.
Actions with other Drugs	Excessive lowering of blood pressure may occur in people taking other blood pressure medication, and especially fluid tablets. As ACE inhibitors prevent the loss of potassium, drugs which add or spare potassium are generally not given at the same time. Ramipril may cause a rise in serum lithium levels.
Pregnancy, Breastfeeding	Ramipril and other ACE inhibitors are not recommended for use in pregnancy as they may cause birth defects. It is not advised for use by nursing mothers.
Special Features, Comments	ACE inhibitors should be used with caution in people with impaired kidney function and in people with narrowing of their heart valves. Older patients may be more susceptible to the medication. Blood tests may be necessary from time to time.

ranitidine

Trade Names	Zantac
How Available	tablet, injection
Drug Group	Anti-ulcer drug
Prescription	Yes
Major Uses	Ranitidine is used for the treatment of ulcers in the stomach and duodenum. Following healing of an ulcer, ranitidine is often continued for a longer period to prevent recurrence. It can also be used to decrease inflammation caused by stomach acid in the esophagus (reflux oesophagitis).
How it Works	Ranitidine is a type of drug called H2 (histamine 2) receptor antagonists. This medication blocks the action of histamine on the cells which produce acid in the stomach. The result is a large drop in the amount of acid produced. This leads to a decrease in inflammation of the linings of the oesophagus, stomach and duodenum, thus for example allowing for the healing of an ulcer.
Usual Dosage	300mg per day as a single dose at night or 150mg twice daily is the usual adult dose for the treatment of peptic ulcer. A maintenance dose of 150mg at night is then used to prevent recurrence of ulcers and this may be continued for 3-12 months or longer. The medication is rarely used in children.
Common Side-Effects	Ranitidine is usually well tolerated. A headache can occur, and allergic reactions are possible. Tiredness, dizziness, nausea, vomiting, diarrhoea and constipation are less common side-effects.
Actions with other Drugs	Unlike cimetidine (another H2 antagonist), ranitidine has no known substantial interactions with other drugs.
Pregnancy, Breastfeeding	Though no known problems have been established, ranitidine is not recommended for use in pregnancy or breastfeeding. It is used only if absolutely necessary.
Special Features, Comments	Alcohol and cigarettes can prevent ulcers from healing, so they are best avoided with ranitidine therapy. This medication should be used with caution in people with impaired kidney function.

roxithromycin

Trade Names	Not available in the UK
How Available	tablet
Drug Group	Antibiotic
Prescription	No
Major Uses	Roxithromycin is most commonly used for the treatment of respiratory tract infections, including infections of the throat, sinuses and tonsils, as well as bronchitis and pneumonia. It can also be used in skin and soft tissue infections and for the treatment of infections caused by Chlamydia.
How it Works	This medication is known as a macrolide and in many ways is similar to erythromycin. It binds with elements within the bacterial cell responsible for the manufacture of protein (ribosomes). At low concentrations this prevents the organism from growing, and at higher concentrations, it kills the bacteria.
Usual Dosage	The usual adult dose is 150mg (one tablet) twice per day before meals. This is usually continued for five days. This medication is not recommended for use in children.
Common Side-Effects	Nausea, vomiting, abdominal pain, diarrhoea, anorexia, flatulence, a rash, and other skin reactions are the commonest side-effects. Other reactions have occurred, but are less likely.
Actions with other Drugs	Use of roxithromycin and theophylline together may increase the level of theophylline. It may also increase the blood levels of disopyramide. Roxithromycin should not be used together with ergotamine.
Pregnancy, Breastfeeding	In general, it is generally safe to use this medication in both pregnancy and breastfeeding.
Special Features, Comments	This medication should be used with caution in people with impaired kidney or liver function.

salbutamol

Trade Names	Aerocrom, Aerolin Autohaler, Asmaven, Salamol, Salbulin, Steri-Neb Salamol, Ventide, Ventodisks, Ventolin, Volmax
How Available	tablet, puffer, rotacaps, nebuliser solution, syrup, injection
Drug Group	Bronchodilator
Prescription	Yes, though the puffer and rotacaps do not require prescription
Major Uses	Salbutamol is used to help prevent and treat asthma. It is also useful in treating breathlessness associated with chronic bronchitis and emphysema. It can be used in pregnancy to prevent premature labour.
How it Works	Salbutamol is a beta-2 sympathomimetic drug. It acts directly on smooth muscle cell receptors in small airways (bronchioles) and the uterus and prevents them from contracting. The drug is related to adrenaline but does not stimulate all of the cell receptors that adrenaline does and thus has far fewer side-effects.
Usual Dosage	This varies greatly depending on the individual. Puffers and other inhaled medications are used every 4-6 hours. Tablets and syrups are given at the same frequency. In children the doses given depend on age and weight.
Common Side-Effects	Anxiety, tremor, headache, dizziness, palpitations and leg cramps are common and are related to the dose of salbutamol used. Side-effects are less common with inhaled medication.
Actions with other Drugs	Salbutamol's effect is diminished by betablockers, which are not commonly used in people with asthma as they make it worse. Other drugs which stimulate the nervous system can make the side-effects of salbutamol worse.
Pregnancy, Breastfeeding	The medication has been used in many women throughout pregnancy with no ill effects on the fetus. It is used therapeutically to prevent premature labour. It may pass into breastmilk, but no ill effects have been demonstrated on infants. It can be used if necessary.
Special Features, Comments	Salbutamol should be given with caution in people with raised blood pressure, coronary artery disease and heart rhythm problems. Diabetics may find that their medications may need to be altered to counteract the effect of salbutamol in raising blood glucose. If the usual dose of the medication does not relieve breathlessness as expected, then medical advice should be sought promptly.

simvastatin

Trade Names	Zocor
How Available	tablet
Drug Group	Lipid lowering drug
Prescription	Yes
Major Uses	Simvastatin is used for the treatment of most types of raised blood cholesterol. It is effective only as long as it is taken and does not eliminate the cause of the raised cholesterol. A low cholesterol diet should be adhered to while the medication is taken.
How it Works	This medication acts by inactivating an enzyme (HMG CoA reductase) which is responsible for one of the first steps in the formation of cholesterol in the liver. (Most of the body's cholesterol is manufactured by the body, rather than taken in with food.) As a result the amount of cholesterol produced by the body is markedly reduced.
Usual Dosage	10-40mg as a single daily dose for adults. It is not recommended for children at present.
Common Side-Effects	Constipation, nausea, flatulence, diarrhoea and headache are the most common side-effects. Other side-effects are much less frequent. Abnormalities in liver function can occur.
Actions with other Drugs	Simvastatin may enhance the effect of oral anti-coagulants. It may cause an inflammation in muscles if used with drugs which suppress the immune system.
Pregnancy, Breastfeeding	It is thought that this group of drugs could cause birth defects, so simvastatin should not be used in pregnancy. It is not recommended for use during breastfeeding.
Special Features, Comments	Adverse effects on liver function are sometimes noted with this drug and blood tests should be performed before treatment and at regular intervals during therapy to assess liver function and also measure response to treatment. Muscle pain and inflammation may occur with the use of HMG CoA reductase inhibitors.

sodium cromoglycate

Trade Names	Aerocrom (with salbutamol), Cromogen, HAY CROM, Intal, Nalcrom, Opticrom, Rynacrom, Steri-Neb Cromogen, Vividrin
How Available	tablet, puffer, nebuliser solution, eye drops
Drug Group	Anti-allergy drug
Prescription	Yes
Major Uses	Sodium chromoglycate is used to prevent allergic reactions. It can be used to prevent asthma if given by puffer or nebuliser. Nasal sprays help prevent hay fever (allergic rhinitis). Eye drops prevent and treat allergic conjunctivitis.
How it Works	This medication prevents the release from cells of substances which give rise to inflammation. It must be used before the substances are released and it is not effective once the allergic process is underway.
Usual Dosage	Two puffs four times a day is the usual dose for the prevention of asthma in both adults and children. Eye drops and nasal preparations are also given four times per day. After a maintenance dose has been established, it may be possible to reduce the dose.
Common Side-Effects	The puffer can cause local irritation to the back of the throat and a dry cough. Dizziness and breathlessness are rare problems. Local irritation to the nose and eye can occur with particular preparations.
Actions with other Drugs	No drug interactions are known.
Pregnancy, Breastfeeding	Sodium chromoglycate has been used during pregnancy and no adverse effects have been established. It is generally recommended as safe. The drug can pass into breastmilk and its safety has not been established in breastfeeding.
Special Features, Comments	Sudden withdrawal of the inhaled medication may lead to a recurrence of asthma.

sodium valproate

Trade Names	Epilim
How Available	tablet, syrup
Drug Group	Anticonvulsant (drug used in epilepsy)
Prescription	Yes
Major Uses	Sodium valproate is used for the prevention of a wide variety of epileptic seizures, either alone, or, if necessary, with other medications.
How it Works	The way this medication works is unknown. It is possible that it may increase the amount of GABA (an inhibitory nerve transmitter substance) in the brain.
Usual Dosage	In adults, 600mg per day is a common starting dose. It is increased depending on the response of the patient to the medication. In children, the dose also depends on age, weight and type of seizures.
Common Side-Effects	Nausea, vomiting, abdominal cramps, drowsiness, unsteadiness and dizziness are common side-effects, although the medication is generally well tolerated. A skin rash can occur. Sodium valproate can impair blood clotting. Impairment of liver function has occurred and is a potentially serious problem.
Actions with other Drugs	Some other anticonvulsants may alter the blood level of sodium valproate. Sodium valproate increases the effect of some antidepressants (MAO inhibitors) and clonazepam.
Pregnancy, Breastfeeding	Women who use anticonvulsant drugs during pregnancy do have an increased chance of birth defects. The chance is about three times normal. If given in the first three months of pregnancy, sodium valproate is suspected of causing damage to the spinal cord. In many cases, there is no alternative but to use anticonvulsants. The potential problems to mother and baby of uncontrolled fitting during pregnancy outweigh the possibility of having an abnormal child. The drug is passed into breast milk and safety in breastfed infants has not been proven.
Special Features, Comments	Due to the sedative effects of the drug, driving and dangerous work should be undertaken with caution. Blood tests at regular intervals are usually taken to assess the level of sodium valproate in the blood. Alcohol can increase the sedative effect of the drug.

sucralfate

Trade Names	Antepsin
How Available	tablet
Drug Group	Anti-ulcer drug
Prescription	Yes
Major Uses	Sucralfate is used to treat ulcers in the stomach and duodenum.
How it Works	When it is swallowed sucralfate (a powder) adheres to the ulcer, protecting the surface cells from further inflammation from gastric acid, pepsin (an enzyme produced by some stomach cells) and bile. This allows ulcer healing to occur, but, like most drugs used to heal ulcers, does not alter the conditions which led to the formation of the ulcer.
Usual Dosage	1g four times per day, one hour before meals and at bedtime, is the usual dose in adults. This is usually continued for six to eight weeks. The medication is not usually given in children and has not been proven safe for their use.
Common Side-Effects	Constipation is the most common side-effect. Others include headache, nausea, an allergic rash, indigestion and dizziness.
Actions with other Drugs	Antacids should not be taken within half an hour of sucralfate, as they may affect binding in the duodenum.
Pregnancy, Breastfeeding	This medication has not been proven safe for use in pregnancy or breastfeeding.
Special Features, Comments	This medication contains aluminium which may accumulate in patients with kidney disease and should be used with caution in such patients. Alcohol and cigarette smoking impair the healing of ulcers so they should be avoided.

sulindac

Trade Names	Clinoril
How Available	tablet
Drug Group	NSAID (non-steroidal anti-inflammatory drug)
Prescription	Yes
Major Uses	Sulindac is a NSAID which is used in a variety of complaints including many types of arthritis and the pain and stiffness associated with inflammation of joints and soft tissues. It can be used to treat gout.
How it Works	This drug prevent the action of substances (prostaglandins) which act on local tissues to produce pain and inflammation.
Usual Dosage	100-400mg per day in divided doses. It is not recommended for use in children.
Common Side-Effects	All NSAIDs produce gastro-intestinal symptoms to some degree. These most commonly are nausea, vomiting and upper abdominal pain. Occasionally an ulcer or bleeding from the stomach or duodenum may occur. (For this reason, people with a history of ulcer disease should not use NSAIDs, including sulindac.) Diarrhoea and constipation can also occur with sulindac. Dizziness, a rash and breathlessness can also occur.
Actions with other Drugs	Use of this drug with aspirin or steroids may increase the chances of peptic ulcer and bleeding. The effect of blood pressure and fluid tablets (diuretics) may be reduced. It may interfere with the effect of anti-coagulant medications. Sulindac may decrease the blood glucose of diabetics taking oral glucose lowering agents.
Pregnancy, Breastfeeding	Sulindac may cause some fetal abnormalities early in pregnancy and may also interfere with fetal blood circulation in the heart late in pregnancy. Thus it is not recommended in pregnancy. It has not been shown to cross over to the infant in breast milk, but its use in breastfeeding should be discussed with your doctor.
Special Features, Comments	Alcohol will increase irritation of the stomach caused by sulindac. It should not be used in people with a history of peptic ulcers. This medication should be given with caution in people with impaired liver function or in people with heart failure. The medication may interfere with clotting and this should be considered before surgery or dental work.

sulphasalazine

Trade Names	Salazopyrin
How Available	tablet, suppository
Drug Group	Drug used for inflammatory disease of the bowel
Prescription	Yes
Major Uses	Sulphasalazine is used to reduce the number and severity of attacks of inflammation caused by two diseases of the bowel known as ulcerative colitis and Crohn's disease. It is sometimes useful in rheumatoid arthritis not responding to other types of medications.
How it Works	The way this medication works is not known. It may interfere with some inflammatory mechanisms in the bowel, or it may act as an anti-inflammatory agent.
Usual Dosage	2-4g daily is the usual adult dose, though the initial dose may be higher. This is usually given in three to four doses. The medication is not usually prescribed in children. Suppositories are given twice per day.
Common Side-Effects	Nausea, loss of appetite and vomiting are the commonest side-effects with this medication. If these are marked then coated tablets should be used to prevent stomach irritation. Other potential side-effects include headache, rashes, joint pain and a rash. It may impair male fertility.
Actions with other Drugs	Sulphasalazine may increase the effects of oral diabetes, drugs, anticoagulants and methotrexate. Digitalis and iron absorption can be reduced by sulphasalazine.
Pregnancy, Breastfeeding	Sulphasalazine has been used in many pregnant women and no adverse effect has been demonstrated. It can be used in pregnancy if necessary. It is not generally advised for use in breastfeeding.
Special Features, Comments	This medication should not be used in people with blood disorders, severe liver or kidney diseases or allergies to either sulphonamide antibiotics or aspirin. If used for a long time, blood and urine tests are usually needed early to detect complications.

sumatriptan

Trade Names	Imigran
How Available	tablet, injection
Drug Group	Anti-migraine drug
Prescription	Yes
Major Uses	Sumatriptan is recommended for the relief of migraine headaches. The injection is also used to treat a migraine variant, known as cluster headaches.
How it Works	This medication is a specific activator of the receptors for 5 hydroxytryptamine1 ($5HT_1$). Most of the these receptors are located in the blood vessels of the brain. Stimulation of these receptors by sumatriptan causes a constriction of these blood vessels. (It is the dilatation of these blood vessels which is thought to be the major cause of migraine in humans.)
Usual Dosage	Injection. The injectable form of the medication comes with an auto injector containing 6mg of sumatriptan. One injection is given, only one other can be given within a 24 hour period. Tablet. The initial dose is a single 100mg tablet. This can be repeated, if necessary, by two further tablets within twenty four hours. It usually takes about 30 minutes for symptoms to respond after a tablet and 15 minutes following an injection. Sumatriptan is not recommended for use in children.
Common Side-Effects	There is commonly discomfort at the site of the injection. Other side-effects of both injection and tablet include a feeling of tingling, heat, heaviness, pressure or tightness in any part of the body; flushing; dizziness and feelings of weakness. Fatigue and drowsiness, nausea and vomiting may occur.
Actions with other Drugs	As both sumatriptan and ergotamine exert similar effects, they should not be given together. Ergotamine should not be used within 6 hours of sumatriptan, and sumatriptan should not be given within 24 hours of ergotamine.
Pregnancy, Breastfeeding	Although no specific problems have been demonstrated, sumatriptan is not recommended in pregnancy or breastfeeding, unless the benefits outweigh the potential risks.

sumatriptan continued

Special Features, Comments

As sumatriptan causes constriction of some blood vessels, it is not recommended for people with known ischaemic heart disease or a history of previous myocardial infarction (heart attack). It is important that the injectable form be given subcutaneously, and not into the vein. People who are driving or operating machinery should be aware of the drowsiness that the medication may cause. People who have had strokes and people who have had heart arrhythmia should not be given sumatriptan.

tamoxifen

Trade Names	Nolvadex, Tamofen
How Available	tablet
Drug Group	Breast cancer drug
Prescription	Yes
Major Uses	Tamoxifen is used for the treatment of breast cancer. It can be used with other treatments such as surgery and radiotherapy to help prevent recurrence of the disease, or to slow the progression of the disease.
How it Works	The medication is known as an anti-oestrogen. It attaches to oestrogen receptors on breast tissue, but unlike normal oestrogen, tamoxifen does not stimulate the growth of breast tissue. As a result the growth of tumours is slowed or even halted.
Usual Dosage	20mg per day is the usual dose, though this may be increased to 40mg.
Common Side-Effects	Specific side-effects which relate to the way this medication works are hot flushes, vaginal bleeding and fluid retention. More general side-effects include nausea, vomiting, light headedness, dizziness and a rash. Some visual problems have occurred with long term use and tamoxifen may interfere with blood clotting.
Actions with other Drugs	This medication may interfere with oral anticoagulant drug treatment.
Pregnancy, Breastfeeding	Tamoxifen is not usually prescribed in either situation or in children.
Special Features, Comments	Abnormal growth of tissue within the uterus may occur. Cystic ovarian swellings are possible in women treated before the menopause. Tamoxifen therapy may interfere with menstruation. Eyesight should be tested at regular intervals if long term treatment is contemplated.

temazepam

Trade Names	Normison
How Available	capsule, tablet
Drug Group	Benzodiazepine
Prescription	Yes
Major Uses	This medication is used for the short-term treatment of sleeplessness. Its effects grow weaker with long periods of continued use.
How it Works	The exact action of this drug and of other drugs in the benzodiazepine group is not known. It works on the central nervous system.
Usual Dosage	10-20mg at night half an hour before retiring is the adult dose. Temazepam is not recommended for use in children.
Common Side-Effects	This medication is quite short-acting and is eliminated from the body quickly. Thus tiredness and drowsiness the day after the medication is taken is rare. Headache and dizziness are the most common side-effects. Blurred vision, confusion and rash are infrequent. Side-effects are more frequent in elderly people.
Actions with other Drugs	Any medication which can cause sedation will add to the sedative side-effects of temazepam. Sleep drugs, antihistamines, anti-depressants, strong analgesics and major tranquillisers will display this additive effect. A reduced tolerance to alcohol is usual.
Pregnancy, Breastfeeding	Temazepam is not recommended in pregnancy. Temazepam can pass into breast milk, so it is not recommended in breastfeeding.
Special Features, Comments	As with other benzodiazepines, there is a potential for dependence with long term use. Also overdosage can occur. Excessive sleepiness and the inability to rouse a person who has access to temazepam should lead to the suspicion of overdosage. Immediate medical attention is necessary. Alcohol should be avoided with temazepam treatment. Driving and hazardous work should be performed cautiously.

tenoxicam

Trade Names	Mobiflex
How Available	tablet
Drug Group	NSAID (non-steroidal anti-inflammatory drug)
Prescription	Yes
Major Uses	Tenoxicam is a NSAID which is used in a variety of complaints including many types of arthritis and the pain and stiffness associated with inflammation of joints and soft tissues.
How it Works	This drug prevents the action of substances (prostaglandins) which act on local tissues to produce pain and inflammation.
Usual Dosage	10-20mg as a once daily dose is usual in adults. It is not recommended for use in children.
Common Side-Effects	All NSAIDs produce gastro-intestinal symptoms to some degree. Nausea and heartburn are the commonest side-effects with tenoxicam. Occasionally an ulcer or bleeding from the stomach or duodenum may occur. (For this reason, people with a history of ulcers should avoid tenoxicam and NSAIDs generally.) Dizziness, headache and a rash are much less likely. Other side-effects have been reported but are thought to be rare, though this medication has not been in use for an extended period of time.
Actions with other Drugs	Tenoxicam may interfere with the action of anti-coagulant drugs. Use of this drug with aspirin or steroids may increase the chances of peptic ulcer. It decreases the effect of frusemide. It may also interfere with lithium levels in the blood. Tenoxicam may increase the action of methotrexate (a drug used for some types of cancers and rheumatoid arthritis) with severe effects on the bone marrow.
Pregnancy, Breastfeeding	Tenoxicam may cause some fetal abnormalities early in pregnancy and may also interfere with the baby's blood circulation in the heart late in pregnancy. Thus it is not recommended in pregnancy. It has not been shown to cross over to the infant in breast milk but its use in breastfeeding should be discussed with your doctor.
Special Features, Comments	This medication should be given with caution in people with impaired liver or kidney function or heart failure. Alcohol will increase the irritation of the stomach caused by tenoxicam. The medication may interfere with clotting and this should be considered before surgery or dental work.

terbinafine

Trade Names	Lamisil
How Available	tablet, cream
Drug Group	Anti-fungal antibiotic
Prescription	Yes
Major Uses	The cream is used for fungal skin infections caused by most types of fungus. Tablets are generally reserved for skin infections which don't respond to topical therapy, for severe infections or for infections where local therapy is difficult. Tablets are also used for fungal nail infections.
How it Works	The medication prevents the formation of a molecule vital for the survival of the fungus.
Usual Dosage	Terbinafine cream is applied once or twice per day, while the usual adult dose of the medication is 250mg per day in a single dose or two doses. The duration of oral treatment depends on the condition being treated and can vary from one week to three months (sometimes six months). Oral terbinafine is not recommended for use in children.
Common Side-Effects	The oral tablet can sometimes cause nausea, flatulence, vomiting, abdominal cramps and discomfort, anorexia and diarrhoea. A rash may occur. Other side-effects are less likely. The cream may cause itchiness, redness or stinging, but this rarely necessitates ceasing treatment.
Actions with other Drugs	The rate of removal of terbinafine from the blood may be decreased by rifampicin and increased by cimetidine. Both these effects are due to interference with the metabolism of terbinafine by the liver. There are no known interactions with the cream.
Pregnancy, Breastfeeding	It is not recommended that oral terbinafine be used in pregnancy or breastfeeding unless thought necessary. There are not thought to be any problems associated with the use of the topical cream.
Special Features, Comments	Terbinafine may occasionally affect liver function, and oral treatment should be used with caution in people with a history of liver problems. A reduced dose of terbinafine may be necessary in these situations and also in people with impaired kidney function.

terbutaline

Trade Names	Bricanyl
How Available	tablet, syrup, injection, puffer, nebuliser solution
Drug Group	Bronchodilator
Prescription	Yes
Major Uses	Terbutaline is used to prevent and treat asthma. It is also useful in treating breathlessness associated with chronic bronchitis and emphysema. It also helps clear mucus from small airways and so is useful in bronchitis.
How it Works	Terbutaline is a beta-2 sympathomimetic drug. It acts directly on smooth muscle cell receptors in small airways (bronchioles) and prevents them from contracting. The drug is related to adrenaline, but does not stimulate all of the cell receptors that adrenaline does, so has far fewer side-effects.
Usual Dosage	The medication is usually given three to four times daily, either orally or via a puffer or nebuliser. Dose depends on severity of the problem treated. In children the doses given depend on age and weight.
Common Side-Effects	Anxiety, tremor, headache, dizziness and palpitations are common and are directly related to the amount of terbutaline used. Side-effects are less common with inhaled medication.
Actions with other Drugs	Terbutaline's therapeutic effects will be decreased by betablockers, though these are not used in people with asthma (they make it worse). Other drugs which stimulate the nervous system can make the side-effects of terbutaline worse. Terbutaline may cause elevated blood pressure if used with some types of antidepressants (MAO inhibitors).
Pregnancy, Breastfeeding	The medication has been used in many women throughout pregnancy with no ill effects on the fetus. It is regarded as safe for use. It may pass into breastmilk, but no ill effects have been demonstrated on infants. It can be used if necessary.
Special Features, Comments	Terbutaline should be given with caution in people with raised blood pressure, coronary artery disease and heart rhythm problems. Diabetics may find that their medications may need to be altered to counteract the effect of terbutaline in raising blood glucose. If the usual dose of the medication does not relieve breathlessness as expected, then medical advice should be sought promptly.

terfenadine

Trade Names	Triludan
How Available	tablet, syrup
Drug Group	Antihistamine (non-sedating)
Prescription	Yes
Major Uses	Terfenadine is used in the treatment of allergic rhinitis (hay fever) in people over six years of age. It is also used in treating some other allergic problems.
How it Works	Antihistamines prevent histamine from reacting with cells and causing local inflammation. Histamine is a naturally occurring substance present in some white blood cells (mast cells). Unlike many antihistamines, terfenadine does not cross over into the central nervous system, so it does not cause drowsiness in the doses normally prescribed.
Usual Dosage	60mg twice per day is the usual adult dose. In children dose depends on age and weight. Terfenadine is not used in children less than six years of age.
Common Side-Effects	Dizziness, headache, dry mouth and a rash can occur with terfenadine, but they are rare. Drowsiness is infrequent.
Actions with other Drugs	The blood levels of some antihistamines can be prolonged with the use of erythromycin, which theoretically could cause a dangerous cardiac rhythm problem. Anticholinergic drugs may add to the effects of terfenadine.
Pregnancy, Breastfeeding	It is not recommended that terfenadine be used in breastfeeding, as safety has not been established. It has been shown to have potential problems in breastfeeding and should not be used.
Special Features, Comments	Overdose should be reported as soon as possible as heart rhythm disturbances are possible.

testosterone

Trade Names	Primoteston, Restandol, Sustanon, Virormone
How Available	tablet, injection, implant beneath the skin
Drug Group	Male sex hormone
Prescription	Yes
Major Uses	Testosterone is the sex hormone produced by the testes in men. (It is also produced in very small amounts in the ovaries in women.) Some males need hormone replacement with testosterone if the testes are not able to produce enough. It can be used to increase libido and may help with some fertility problems in men. It is sometimes used in women to treat breast cancer and thin bones in women. Testosterone may be used as a male contraceptive, though this use is not widespread at present.
How it Works	Testosterone acts on a wide variety of cells and any cell that normally responds to the hormone will respond to the introduced medication.
Usual Dosage	This depends on the problem treated. Tablets are given every day, injections every week to a month and implants changed two to three times yearly.
Common Side-Effects	In males, the common side-effects include an increased frequency of erections, difficulty in passing urine, salt and water retention and short stature (if the drug is given before the end of puberty). In women, unusual hair growth and a deepening of the voice can occur.
Actions with other Drugs	Testosterone can increase the effect of anti-coagulants and also the effect of oral blood glucose lowering drugs.
Pregnancy, Breastfeeding	The medication is not intended to be used in pregnant women. Birth defects can occur. Likewise the medication is not recommended for use in breastfeeding women.
Special Features, Comments	Special care must be taken if testosterone is used in people with heart, liver or kidney disease, epilepsy or migraine. Blood tests may be necessary at regular intervals to ensure that any biochemical irregularities are corrected early.

tetracycline

Trade Names	Achromycin, Deteclo, Sustamycin, Tetrabid, Tetrachel
How Available	tablet, liquid
Drug Group	Tetracycline antibiotic
Prescription	Yes
Major Uses	Tetracycline is an antibiotic effective against a wide variety of bacteria. It is used for ear, throat and respiratory tract infections as well as some types of pneumonia. It can be used for some sexually transmitted diseases and is effective in prostate and skin infections. Its antibacterial activity is used to treat acne.
How it Works	This drug acts by preventing the formation of protein within bacteria. It prevents bacteria from growing, rather than killing the bacteria.
Usual Dosage	0.5-2g per day in divided doses depending on the severity and type of problem treated is the adult dose range. The drug is not usually given to children less than eight years of age.
Common Side-Effects	Nausea, vomiting and diarrhoea are the most common side-effects, made more common because this antibiotic should not be taken with food (as absorption is decreased). A rash, especially after sun exposure, can occur. Many other potential side-effects can occur, but these are much less frequent.
Actions with other Drugs	Antacids can decrease the absorption of tetracycline. Some epilepsy drugs can decrease its effect. Tetracycline can interfere with the oral contraceptive pill, and anti-coagulant drugs. Tetracycline may also interfere with the action of penicillin and is not usually given at the same time. Iron tablets can reduce the effect of tetracycline.
Pregnancy, Breastfeeding	This group of drugs can interfere with the growth and development of teeth in the fetus, and in children less than eight years of age. This causes discoloured teeth. It causes retarded bone growth as well. It is not recommended for use by pregnant or breastfeeding women.
Special Features, Comments	Alcohol and tetracyclines can both cause irritation to the stomach, so they should not be used together.

theophylline

Trade Names	Franol, Lasma, Nuelin, Slo-Phyllin, Theo-Dur, Uniphyllin Continus
How Available	tablets, sustained release tablets, syrup
Drug Group	Bronchodilator
Prescription	Yes
Major Uses	Theophylline is used in the treatment of asthma. It is also useful in treating breathlessness associated with chronic bronchitis and emphysema. Occasionally, it is given to premature infants in order to stimulate breathing.
How it Works	Theophylline acts within smooth muscle cells lining the small airways and blood vessels of the lung and interferes with the breakdown of a substance (cyclic AMP) thus preventing contraction of the muscle cell.
Usual Dosage	400-600mg daily in divided doses every six hours or every twelve hours (with sustained release preparations). In children the doses given depend on age and weight.
Common Side-Effects	Nausea, vomiting, palpitations, tremor and agitation are the commonest side-effects. Other side-effects are rare.
Actions with other Drugs	Erythromycin and cimetidine may increase the level of theophylline in the blood. Some drugs used for epilepsy may decrease theophylline levels.
Pregnancy, Breastfeeding	This medication has been used in pregnancy and no adverse effects have been established. It is generally considered safe for use. Theophylline does pass into breastmilk and its elimination may be slow, especially in premature infants. It is used only if potential benefits outweigh risks.
Special Features, Comments	Theophylline should be given with caution to people with known heart and blood pressure problems. Heart, lung, kidney and liver problems decrease the rate of elimination of the drug. A higher dose of theophylline may be necessary in smokers. There is a relatively small difference between therapeutic and toxic blood levels of this medication, and an overdose can occur relatively easily. This can be a serious problem. The side-effects listed above are early indications of this potential problem. Immediate medical advice should be sought.

thioridazine

Trade Names	Melleril
How Available	tablet, syrup
Drug Group	Psychiatric drug
Prescription	Yes
Major Uses	Thioridazine is known as a major tranquilliser of the phenothiazine type. It is used to treat mental health problems such as schizophrenia, mania, short term confusion and very aggressive behaviour. It also has many other uses in psychiatry. It may also be of use in treating intractable pain.
How it Works	The phenothiazines have many activities in the brain and the chemicals which transmit messages in the brain. Their major action is probably reducing the activity of one of these neurotramsmitters, dopamine.
Usual Dosage	This varies considerably from 50mg to 400mg per day. The medication is not usually prescribed in children.
Common Side-Effects	Tiredness, dry mouth, stuffy nose, light-headedness and dizziness are common side-effects. Blurred vision may occur. It causes less movement problems than other phenothiazines. In low doses, movement problems and longer term involuntary movement disorders are uncommon.
Actions with other Drugs	Any medication which can cause sedation will add to the sedative side-effects of thioridazine. Sleep drugs, antihistamines, benzodiazepines, antidepressants, strong analgesics and major tranquillisers will display this additive effect as will alcohol. Thioridazine may decrease the beneficial effects of drugs used for Parkinson's disease. Other drugs which have anticholinergic properties may add to the side-effects of thioridazine.
Pregnancy, Breastfeeding	After birth, babies of women who have taken thioridazine may have movement disorders. Thioridazine is generally not used in pregnancy or breastfeeding, unless absolutely necessary.
Special Features, Comments	The medication may need to be stopped before surgery. Driving and hazardous work should be performed with great caution. Alcohol should be avoided while this medication is used. Routine blood tests may need to be performed as liver function can be affected with long term use.

thyroxine

Trade Names	Eltroxin
How Available	tablet
Drug Group	Thyroid hormone
Prescription	Yes
Major Uses	Thyroxine is identical to the hormone produced by the thyroid gland. It is used if the thyroid gland is under functioning (hypothyroidism). It can be used in some types of goitre (enlargement of the thyroid gland) and in some thyroid cancers. It is sometimes used with antithyroid drugs to stop goitres from forming and in a type of over-active thyroid disease, Hashimoto's disease.
How it Works	Thyroxine works in the same way as the natural hormone, increasing the amount of the active hormone (tri-iodothyronine) to tissues and feeding back to the brain information about thyroid hormone production.
Usual Dosage	50-200 micrograms is the average daily dose in adults. Children require a lower dose according to weight and age.
Common Side-Effects	If given in the correct dose thyroxine is well tolerated. However, if excess amounts are given, then anxiousness, diarrhoea, sweating, and weight loss can occur. Similar, but more prominent side-effects are possible if an overdose of thyroxine is taken.
Actions with other Drugs	Thyroxine can reduce the effect of blood glucose lowering medications and digoxin. Some cholesterol lowering drugs can lower thyroxine absorption. Thyroxine may interfere with oral anticoagulant therapy. Many drugs can interfere with tests for thyroid function and give an incorrect assessment of the effect of thyroxine therapy.
Pregnancy, Breastfeeding	Thyroxine has been used extensively during pregnancy and in breastfeeding and is generally regarded as safe to use in both.
Special Features, Comments	Blood tests should be performed at regular intervals to ensure that the amount of thyroxine given is appropriate. Care should be taken in giving thyroxine to people with severely impaired thyroid function, heart disease or decreased adrenal gland function.

tiaprofenic acid

Trade Names	Surgam
How Available	tablet
Drug Group	NSAID (non-steroidal anti-inflammatory drug)
Prescription	Yes
Major Uses	Tiaprofenic acid is a NSAID which is used in a variety of complaints including many types of arthritis and the pain and stiffness pain associated with inflammation of joints and soft tissues.
How it Works	This drug prevents the action of substances (prostaglandins) which act on local tissues to produce pain and inflammation.
Usual Dosage	200-600mg per day in two doses is the usual adult dose. This drug is not recommended for use in children.
Common Side-Effects	All NSAIDs produce gastro-intestinal symptoms to some degree. Indigestion, nausea, heartburn, abdominal pain, flatulence and diarrhoea are common side-effects. Occasionally an ulcer, or bleeding from the stomach or duodenum may occur. (For this reason, people with a history of ulcers should avoid tiaprofenic acid and NSAIDs in general). Dizziness, a rash, hot flushes are less likely. Many other side-effects have been reported, but are rare.
Actions with other Drugs	Tiaprofenic acid may interfere with the effect of anticoagulant drugs, phenytoin, lithium, sulphur based antibiotics and some drugs used to treat diabetes. It may also interfere with the effect of another drug sometimes used to treat arthritis, methotrexate. Use of tiaprofenic acid with aspirin or steroids may increase the chances of peptic ulcer. The drug may interfere with the action of diuretic tablets.
Pregnancy, Breastfeeding	This medication does cross into the fetus during pregnancy. It is not recommended for use in pregnancy or breastfeeding.
Special Features, Comments	This medication should be given with caution in people with impaired liver or kidney function or in people with heart failure. Alcohol will increase the irritation of the stomach caused by tiaprofenic acid. The medication should be used with caution in the elderly. It may interfere with blood clotting, which should be considered before surgery or dental work.

timolol

Trade Names	Betim, Blocadren, Glaucol, Moducren, Prestim, Timoptol
How Available	tablet, eye drops
Drug Group	Betablocker
Prescription	Yes
Major Uses	Timolol is most commonly used to treat raised blood pressure. It may also be used to treat angina (pain from inadequate oxygen supply to the heart muscle). It is sometimes used after a heart attack to prevent further damage to the heart muscle. Some disturbances of heart rhythm may be treated with timolol. It can also be used to prevent migraine headaches. The drops treat some types of glaucoma (raised pressure within the eye).
How it Works	The means by which timolol decreases blood pressure is not known. It decreases heart rate, and this is one of the reasons it is effective in angina, but does not explain its ability to lower blood pressure. It has a direct effect on an area of the heart responsible for the rate at which the heart beats, controlling some rhythm disturbances.
Usual Dosage	Eye drops, twice daily. Tablets, 20-50mg daily.
Common Side-Effects	Tiredness, dizziness and light-headedness are the most common side-effects with the tablets. The drops may cause blurred vision, eye irritation and headache.
Actions with other Drugs	Calcium antagonists may reduce heart rate if given with betablockers. Some types antidepressants react adversely with timolol.
Pregnancy, Breastfeeding	Timolol has been used for the treatment of raised blood pressure in pregnant women without recognised adverse effects. It can lower the fetal heart rate, which may be important at delivery. It is not suggested for use by nursing mothers.
Special Features, Comments	It can be dangerous to withdraw this drug suddenly as a rapid rise in blood pressure or increase in heart oxygen consumption may occur. People with diseased arteries to the legs may have worsen symptoms if timolol is used. Unstable diabetics should avoid timolol as it may mask signs of a low blood glucose level. People with asthma or chronic bronchitis should avoid timolol. It may make their problems worse. The drug may need to be stopped before a general anaesthetic is given. An overdose of this medication can be serious and immediate medical attention should be sought.

tolbutamide

Trade Names	Rastinon
How Available	tablet
Drug Group	Oral antidiabetic drug (sulphonylurea)
Prescription	Yes
Major Uses	Tolbutamide is useful in NIDDM (non-insulin dependent diabetes mellitus), if diet alone cannot give adequate blood glucose control. It is vital that a diabetic diet is followed, while the medication is used, if it is to be effective.
How it Works	Sulphonylurea drugs lower blood glucose by stimulating the pancreas to produce more insulin (the hormone mostly responsible for increasing uptake of glucose into cells).
Usual Dosage	500mg-2g usually in divided doses is usual for adults. NIDDM does not occur in children, so the medication is not prescribed.
Common Side-Effects	The most common and most worrying side-effect of oral antidiabetic drugs is that they may lower blood glucose excessively (hypoglycaemia). The warning signs of this are confusion, feeling faint and weak, sweating and tremor. It should be suspected if any of these symptoms develop. Carbohydrate in the form of a sweet biscuit or glucose sweet should be given immediately
Actions with other Drugs	Other drugs given at the same time can lower blood glucose and make hypoglycaemia more likely. These drugs include alcohol, betablockers, other blood glucose lowering agents, aspirin, sulphonamide and tetracycline antibiotics as well as chloramphenicol and anti-coagulant drugs. Some other drugs may decrease the effect of sulphonylureas. These include steroids, oestrogens, some fluid tablets and others.
Pregnancy, Breastfeeding	Control of diabetes in pregnancy is usually achieved most effectively with insulin, so oral antidiabetic drugs are not generally used. It is not known whether they enter breastmilk but they are not generally used in nursing mothers.
Special Features, Comments	Regular blood and/or urine testing for glucose is necessary. Tolbutamide may cause metabolic problems if the body is under severe stress e.g. after physical trauma. Overdosage with tolbutamide may lead to unconsciousness and requires immediate medical treatment.

tranylcypromine

Trade Names	Parnate, Parnstelin
How Available	tablet
Drug Group	Antidepressant (MAO inhibitor)
Prescription	Yes

Major Uses
Tranylcypromine is a member of a group of drugs known as mono-amine oxidase inhibitors (MAO inhibitors). These medications are used to treat severe depression and are very effective at improving mood, increasing activity and appetite. They are usually used if other medications with fewer potential side-effects are ineffective. Tranylcypromine usually takes two to three weeks to exert its full effect.

How it Works
The action of MAO inhibitors is widespread. It stops the break down of a number of important nerve transmission substances, by blocking the action of the enzyme monoamine oxidase. It may also act in other ways as well.

Usual Dosage
20mg per day is the usual starting dose. This is increased to 30mg or until the desired antidepressant effects result. The medication is then decreased until the lowest dose maintaining effect is reached. Tranylcypromine is not recommended for use in children.

Common Side-Effects
The most common adverse reaction with tranylcypromine is insomnia. In fact, a mild sleep drug may be needed as well. Other common side-effects include dizziness, dry mouth, lightheadedness, an excessive fall in blood pressure when standing, constipation and weakness. A rash, nausea and vomiting and a headache may occur. Inflammation of the liver is rare. Agitation, euphoria and agitation can occur.

Actions with other Drugs
The major problem with the use of MAO Inhibitors is that they interact with many other medications and even some foods e.g. cheeses, Vegemite and red wine. The most serious adverse reaction consists of a sudden and potentially dangerous increase in blood pressure. Many medications, even cough remedies and non-prescription drugs may cause this reaction. It is imperative that medical advice be sought before any additional medication is taken. Other antidepressant medications should not be given during, or for a week after stopping tranylcypromine treatment, as other potentially serious problems may occur.

tranylcypromine continued

Pregnancy, Breastfeeding

This medication is not recommended for use in pregnant or breastfeeding women, though no specific problems have been established. As some drugs used in childbirth may cause severe interactions with tranylcypromine, it is usually stopped two weeks before the intended delivery date.

Special Features, Comments

This medication should not be used in people with epilepsy, raised blood pressure or reduced arterial flow to the heart or brain. Tranylcypromine should be stopped a week before any planned general anaesthetic. Red wine can cause a serious reaction with tranylcypromine. Other alcohol should be avoided. Driving and dangerous work should be undertaken with caution. Overdose with tranylcypromine is possible, with sweating and fever common symptoms. If suspected, immediate medical advice should be sought.

tretinoin

Trade Names	Retin-A
How Available	cream, gel
Drug Group	Acne treatment
Prescription	Yes, generally
Major Uses	Tretinoin is used for the treatment of acne of all levels of severity.
How it Works	The general effect of treinoin is to increase the growth and proliferation of skin cells. This results in diminished thickness of the upper layers of the skin and thus a beneficial effect on acne.
Usual Dosage	The medication is usually applied on a single occasion at night before retiring, though some people require less intensive therapy. It is often possible to maintain an established response with treatment less than once per day.
Common Side-Effects	Most common side-effects are redness, irritation and stinging of the skin. This often occurs at the beginning of a treatment course. The skin may become swollen, blistered or crusted. Some people have a heightened susceptibility to sunlight while using tretinoin. A temporary increase or decrease in skin pigmentation may occur. Local allergic reactions may occur. Occasionally there may be an alteration in liver function.
Actions with other Drugs	As the drug is usually used in isolation, few interactions have been reported. Usually a rest period between the use of other topical preparations and the use of tretinoin is recommended to limit potential problems.
Pregnancy, Breastfeeding	Tretinoin is generally thought to be safe to use in recommended doses in pregnancy and breastfeeding.
Special Features, Comments	Use of sun screens, and avoidance of the sun is recommended while using tretinoin therapy, due to increased light sensitivity. Weather extremes of wind and cold may also cause increased skin irritation. Tretinoin should be kept away from the eyes, mouth and nose. The medication may result in inflammation to skin affected by eczema.

triazolam

Trade Names	Not yet available in the UK
How Available	tablet
Drug Group	Benzodiazepine
Prescription	No
Major Uses	This medication is used to induce sleep. It is used to correct short term disturbances in sleep patterns.
How it Works	The exact action of this drug and of other drugs in the benzodiazepine group is not known, but it is thought to depress the activity in that part of the brain which controls emotion. It works on the central nervous system. This medication is very short acting, and is not useful for treating anxiety as are many other benzodiazepines.
Usual Dosage	0.125-0.5mg at night is the range of doses that adults usually take at night before retiring. Triazolam is not recommended for children less than eighteen years of age.
Common Side-Effects	Drowsiness, sedation, lightheadedness, headache, impaired co-ordination, nervousness, nausea and lethargy are all common side-effects with triazolam therapy. Other side-effects are possible, but occur much less commonly. Elderly people are more likely to suffer from adverse reactions.
Actions with other Drugs	Any medication which can cause sedation will add to the sedative side-effects of triazolam. Sleep drugs, antihistamines, antidepressants, strong analgesics, other benzodiazepines and major tranquillisers will display this effect as will alcohol. Erythromycin and cimetidine may increase the effect of triazolam.
Pregnancy, Breastfeeding	This medication is not recommended for use in pregnancy or breastfeeding.
Special Features, Comments	Driving and dangerous work should not be undertaken while this medication is active. Even activities such as walking across a busy street may be dangerous, because of impaired judgement. This medication may cause withdrawal symptoms if removed from the system abruptly, and changes in dose should only be made on doctor's advice. A reduced dose may be necessary in people with severe liver or kidney problems.

trimipramine

Trade Names	Surmontil
How Available	tablet
Drug Group	Tricyclic antidepressant
Prescription	Yes
Major Uses	This medication is used for the treatment of depression and also helps to induce sleep. The antidepressant effects start after two to three weeks of treatment.
How it Works	The exact mode of action of this group of drugs on the central nervous system is not known.
Usual Dosage	50-100mg in one dose two hours before bedtime.
Common Side-Effects	When trimipramine is started or the dose increased the following side-effects are very common. They include drowsiness, dry mouth, sweating, blurred vision, constipation and difficulty passing urine. Other side-effects have been reported in individuals. Confusion may occur in elderly patients.
Actions with other Drugs	All drugs, including alcohol, which have a sedative effect will have an additive effect on trimipramine. Sleep drugs, antihistamines, other antidepressants, strong analgesics, benzodiazepines and major tranquillisers are the most common examples. Trimipramine and other tricyclic antidepressants should not be used at the same time as another type of antidepressant (MAO inhibitors) as occasionally very serious side-effects may occur. Trimipramine may reduce the effect of some blood pressure reducing drugs. Smoking and barbiturates can reduce the antidepressant effect of this drug.
Pregnancy, Breastfeeding	Safe use of this medication in pregnant women has not been established. Its use should be avoided if possible. Nursing mothers should also avoid the drug as it can pass into breast milk.
Special Features, Comments	All tricyclic antidepressants including trimipramine can have serious consequences if an overdose is taken as this will have a profound effect on the heart. Dizziness, blurred vision, dry mouth, agitation, convulsions and lack of arousal should give rise to suspicion of overdosage. Immediate medical attention is imperative. Due to its sedative properties, it is important not to drive or perform hazardous work until the effect of the drug is established. Alcohol will increase sedation.

verapamil

Trade Names	Berkatens, Cordilox, Securon, Univer
How Available	tablet, slow-release tablet, injection
Drug Group	Calcium channel blocker
Prescription	Yes
Major Uses	Verapamil is most commonly used to treat raised blood pressure. In addition, it can be used to prevent angina (pain in the chest due to insufficient oxygen supply to the heart muscle). Due to its action on the conduction system in the heart, verapamil is employed to slow down the heart rate in some arrhythmias.
How it Works	Calcium channel blockers are thought to prevent the flow of calcium through the smooth muscle cell membranes which line small arteries. This decreases blood pressure, increases flow through the arteries and prevents spasm of the walls of arteries (which occurs in the heart in some attacks of angina). Verapamil slows the conduction of the heart's electrical impulse at a site called the AV node.
Usual Dosage	80-480mg per day in divided doses (except for the once per day slow-release tablets) is the usual adult dose. It is not generally used in children.
Common Side-Effects	Constipation, headache, dizziness, flushing and ankle swelling are common side-effects with verapamil. They usually occur at the start of treatment and disappear or decrease with time.
Actions with other Drugs	Verapamil increases the effects of drugs which lower blood pressure. Beta-blockers can lead to a serious slowing of heart rate if used with verapamil. Other medications which decrease the contractile power of the heart muscle should be used with caution with verapamil. Verapamil may increase the blood level of digoxin.
Pregnancy, Breastfeeding	This medication is generally not prescribed in either pregnancy or breastfeeding. It may inhibit labour and can theoretically cause birth defects.
Special Features, Comments	Verapamil should be used cautiously in people with heart failure. Some heart rhythm problems should not be treated with verapamil. Alcohol may accentuate the blood pressure lowering properties of the drug and may add to side-effects.

warfarin

Trade Names	Marevan, Warfarin
How Available	tablet
Drug Group	Oral anticoagulant
Prescription	Yes

Major Uses

Warfarin is used to prevent and treat blood clots within blood vessels. It can be used to treat clots in the veins of the leg, and prevent clots in vessels in the lungs (pulmonary emboli). If the heart is enlarged or beating irregularly, warfarin may be of use in preventing clots from forming on the walls of the heart chambers. People with artificial heart valves usually take warfarin long-term. Often warfarin therapy is begun in hospital and may follow on from treatment with another drug, heparin.

How it Works

This medication works by blocking the action of vitamin K in the liver. This leads to a decrease in the formation of some clotting factors, hence clots are much less likely to form.

Usual Dosage

When warfarin is started, the full anti-clotting effect does not take place for two to three days. Often a higher than normal daily dose is given for the first day or two of treatment. Once stable, adult doses are usually 1-10mg. Strict monitoring of the clotting capacity of the blood is necessary. This is most commonly achieved using a blood test called the prothrombin ratio. This is normally kept in a therapeutic range of 2-4 for people on warfarin treatment. Warfarin dosage varies greatly with each person and also time. Doses in children are also highly individual, though lower.

Common Side-Effects

The most potentially serious side-effect of warfarin therapy is abnormal bleeding. Black, tarry bowel motions are often the first indicator of a bleed from the gastro-intestinal tract though any indication of bleeding from any part of the body should be noted. Bleeding can occur even if the medication is in the therapeutic range. Any unusual symptoms should be reported to a doctor. Other side-effects include fever, nausea, diarrhoea, hair loss and allergic reactions.

warfarin continued

Actions with other Drugs

Many drugs are known to increase or decrease the anticoagulant effect of warfarin. These can even include some medications which can be purchased without prescription. It is vital that medical advice be sought before any other drug is taken. If another medication is introduced, a change to warfarin dose will often to necessary. Aspirin may prolong the effect of warfarin and may increase the chances of bleeding.

Pregnancy, Breastfeeding

Oral anticoagulants cause fetal abnormalities and fetal death and should not be used in pregnancy. If an oral anticoagulant is needed in breastfeeding, then warfarin is preferred to phenindione. In most women, a therapeutic dose of warfarin will not pass into the breastmilk.

Special Features, Comments

Regular blood tests are vital to the long term successful use of warfarin. Warfarin needs to be stopped or other anticoagulant medications used before surgery or dental work, to avoid excessive bleeding. Alcohol may alter the dose of warfarin needed. It is important that diet and the level of physical exercise is consistent while on warfarin therapy as both of these factors may influence coagulation. Any illness such as infection, heart disease, recent surgery or liver disease will either increase or decrease the dose of warfarin needed. Warfarin should not be used in people with bleeding disorders e.g. haemophilia, in people with ulcers or bleeding areas in the gastro-intestinal or urinary tract. It should not be used in people with severe liver or kidney disease.

zidovudine (formerly known as azidothymidine or AZT)

Trade Names	Retrovir
How Available	tablet
Drug Group	Anti-viral antibiotic
Prescription	Yes
Major Uses	Zidovudine is a medication used in people who have AIDS (acquired immunodeficiency syndrome). The drug is used to slow the progression of the disease. It has been shown to prevent weight loss and decrease the number of infections that AIDS patients develop. In addition, it can slow the progression of AIDS within the central nervous system. Some doctors believe that it can be beneficial before overt infections occur.
How it Works	This drug acts by interfering with the multiplication of HIV (human immunodeficiency virus). It does this by stopping the virus from forming an image of its genetic material, which is a necessary step in its reproduction. (Specifically, it inhibits an enzyme known as DNA-polymerase.)
Usual Dosage	200mg is usually given every four hours, i.e. 6 daily doses. Lower doses also may be effective with less side-effects. A decreased dose is given to children, depending on age and weight.
Common Side-Effects	The most worrying side-effect of zidovudine is the impairment of the blood forming cells in the bone marrow. This impairment is directly related to the dose of the medication given. Many side-effects are possible with the drug and include nausea, vomiting, tiredness, muscle aches, headache, breathlessness and impaired liver function.
Actions with other Drugs	Probenecid may impair excretion of the drug. Other drugs which decrease kidney or liver function should be given with caution, as should all medications which can depress blood cell production.
Pregnancy, Breastfeeding	Fetal abnormalities have not been demonstrated with this medication. The drug is recommended for use in pregnant women only if there is a clear benefit. It is not advised for use in breastfeeding, bottle-feeding is preferred.
Special Features, Comments	This medication is given only under strict supervision in hospitals or in specialised AIDS treatment units. Regular blood tests are needed to assess the effect of the drug on the HIV virus and the blood.

Glossary

Acromegaly An illness in which increased amounts of growth hormone are secreted from the base of the brain (the pituitary gland).

Adrenal gland This gland sits directly above each kidney. It is responsible for producing two types of hormones, adrenalin and noradrenalin, and steroid hormones (glucocorticoids and mineralocorticoids).

Amoeba A general term for advanced types of single celled organisms. They can cause many illnesses, though the most common are diarrhoeal illnesses.

Anaemia This term is used when the amount of haemoglobin in the blood is low. There are many types of anaemia.

Anticholinergic Any drug which has anticholinergic properties blocks one arm of the nervous system (the parasympathetic nervous system). This leads to some characteristic effects such as sedation, dry mouth, constipation, difficulty urinating and blurred vision.

Antihypertensive Any medication which is used therapeutically to lower blood pressure.

Aplastic anaemia A type of anaemia in which blood cell production in the bone marrow is suppressed. This may involve white cells, red cells, platelets or all three.

Atherosclerosis A medical condition in which fatty material and cholesterol are laid down on the inside of arteries. If the blockage is severe, vital tissues are deprived of oxygen.

Bacteria Very small single celled organisms, surrounded by a cell membrane and cell wall. Bacteria are responsible for many of the infections for which antibiotics are used.

Barbiturates Once used for sedation and as sleep inducing drugs, barbiturates are no longer commonly prescribed in Australia. They have an addiction potential and may cause serious breathing problems if taken in overdosage.

Beta 2 One arm of the nervous system. The sympathetic nervous system has two types of receptors, alpha and beta. Beta receptors can be further divided into beta 1 and beta 2. Beta 2 receptors are only found in the lung and uterus, so drugs which stimulate them alone help relieve asthma and prevent premature labour without excessive side-effects.

Blood level The level of a particular substance in serum. (Serum is whole blood which has been allowed to clot in a test-tube.)

Bronchodilator Any substance which dilates the small passages which lead to the periphery of the lung.

Chrohn's disease This is a disease of unknown cause, leading to inflammation of the bowel.

Chronic bronchitis A disease in which there is diffuse inflammation of the air passages in the lungs, leading to decreased uptake of oxygen by the lungs and increased mucus production.

Corticosteroid A type of hormone produced by the adrenal gland. In the body these hormones dampen down inflammation and help the body cope with the stress of injury or trauma.

Duodenum The stomach discharges food onwards into the duodenum, the first part of the small bowel. It is about 12cm long.

Electrolytes Sodium, chloride, potassium and bicarbonate are the most important electrolytes or salt components within the blood stream.

Emphysema Diffuse damage to very small airways and the structural material of the lung, leading to diminished transfer of oxygen into the blood.

Enzyme A protein molecule which speeds up specific chemical reactions, without itself changing. These are widespread within cells, on cell membranes and also in the blood and blood cells.

Fungus A type of organism responsible for many infections. There are many types, causing infections of the skin, vagina, mouth and gastrointestinal tract as well as some rare but serious infections throughout the body.

Generic The generic name of a drug is the name of the active ingredient, as distinct from the name given to a particular product (which contains the drug), by a manufacturer. A doctor may prescribe a medication by product name or generic name.

Growth hormone One of a number of hormones secreted from the pituitary gland at the base of the brain. Diminished secretion leads to retarded growth, increased secretion to acromegaly.

Haemolytic anaemia A type of anaemia in which red cells are actually destroyed within the bloodstream.

Hepatitis Any condition in which there is an inflammation of the liver.

Histamine A substance produced in the body which causes local inflammation when released. It is responsible for many of the manifestations of allergic reactions.

Histamine H2 antagonist Histamine acts on the receptors of some cells in the stomach to stimulate the release of acid. These receptors are called H2 receptors. Some drugs, H2 receptor antagonists, block the action of histamine, so reducing stomach acid production.

Hormone A substance which is released from one area of the body and travels via the bloodstream to another, where it exerts its effect.

Hypertension Elevated blood pressure. The exact level at which blood pressure is deemed to be elevated depends on a person's age, though as a general rule for adults 140mm.Hg is the upper systolic limit and 90mm.Hg is the upper diastolic limit.

Interaction Altered reaction of the body to one drug when another is taken as well.

Jaundice A build up of bilirubin (bile pigment) in the blood, as a result of the liver's inability to excrete it effectively. This leads to a yellow discolouration of the eyes and skin.

Liver function tests These are tests for the blood levels of bilirubin and also some enzymes normally present in liver cells. Abnormalities point to malfunction or inflammation of the liver.

MAO inhibitor Mono-amine oxidase inhibitor. A type of antidepressant medication. Due to its widespread actions within the body, these medications interact with a large number of prescription and non-prescription drugs.

Neurotransmitter A substance released by a nerve cell which allows the transmission of a signal to a nearby nerve cell.

Obsessive compulsive disorders A psychiatric condition in which a person performs tasks repeatedly and unnecessarily e.g. washing their hands.

Oesophagus The oesophagus leads from the back of the throat to the stomach. The lower end may be affected by a reflux of acid from the stomach.

Pancreas An organ of the body which secretes substances into the small bowel to aid digestion and also produces important hormones such as insulin and glucagon.

Parasympathetic Referring to one arm of the nervous system, the parasympathetic nervous system. This is responsible for some aspects of breathing, digestion and many other functions. In general, it does the opposite of the sympathetic nervous system.

Parkinson's disease A disorder of movement. This disease is characterised by a tremor and also a difficulty in initiating movement.

Peptic ulcer Any ulcer of the gastro-intestinal tract which is caused by irritation from stomach juices. They not only occur in the stomach, but also in the duodenum and oesophagus.

Pituitary gland A gland at the base of the brain which releases hormones in response to stimuli higher in the brain (the hypothalamus).

Platelet A small component of blood which is responsible for one type of clotting within the bloodstream.

Potassium An important electrolyte in cells and the blood. Small changes in blood levels of potassium can have profound effects on muscle and heart function.

Prolactin A hormone secreted by the pituitary gland. Prolactin is important in the initiation and maintenance of breastfeeding.

Prophylactic A medication taken as a preventative measure.

Raynaud's disease A condition in which the extremities of the body react excessively to cold, resulting in an uncomfortable reduction in the amount of blood circulating to the fingers and toes.

Receptor A protein molecule (most commonly on the surface of a cell) which reacts to a substance which stimulates it. This leads to further biochemical changes within the cell itself.

Rheumatoid arthritis A specific type of arthritis which may lead to destruction of joints. The type and severity of rheumatoid arthritis varies considerably.

Rotacap A small gelatin capsule of a bronchodilator substance which is used in a rotahaler as an alternative to a puffer.

Schizophrenia A complex psychiatric illness characterised by altered thoughts and unusual phenomena such as auditory hallucinations.

Skin patch (transdermal patch) Some medications can be absorbed into the bloodstream through the skin. If this is the case, sustained levels of the medication can be obtained by use of a transdermal patch.

SLE (systemic lupus erythematosus) This is a condition characterised by inflammation of many tissues, including joints, skin and possibly arteries, kidney and other tissues.

Suppository A medication which is inserted into the rectum. It may be absorbed or act locally (e.g. to treat haemorrhoids).

Sympathomimetic Referring to one arm of the nervous system, the sympathetic nervous system. Generally, this exerts an opposite effect to the parasympathetic nervous system. It is responsible for regulating many body functions, including heart rate, breathing and digestion.

Thyroid gland A gland in the neck which secretes thyroid hormones, responsible for increasing the body's metabolic rate and the rate of utilisation of energy stores.

Tolerance This occurs when the body becomes accustomed to the therapeutic effect of a drug. More may be needed to achieve the desired effect.

Topical Applied to the skin or membrane, directly on to the affected area.

Toxic Poisonous. Many medications are poisonous if very high doses are taken deliberately or inadvertently. Some medications are toxic at doses not much higher than therapeutic doses.

Triglycerides A type of fat. Triglycerides are the most common types of fat in the body and are also present in the blood. They are a major source of energy, but not nearly as important as cholesterol in the formation of atherosclerosis.

Ulcerative colitis A disease of unknown cause which leads to inflammation, mostly of the large bowel.

Uric acid A substance which is present in the body. Excessive amounts of uric acid may crystalise in joints causing an inflammation known as gout.

Urinary tract The organs responsible for the production and excretion of urine. These are the kidneys, ureters, bladder and urethra.

Vaccine A substance which stimulates the immune system to produce a response to a specific infection without actually exposing the body to the true infection.

Vasodilator Any drug which dilates arterial blood vessels.

Virus Viruses are infective agents which are very small and are unable to grow and multiply unless they invade the cell of another organism. Viruses are very common. To date, only a few antibiotics exist which are effective against them.

Wilson's disease A rare disease in which copper accumulates in the liver and brain. It can lead to liver disease and retarded mental development in children.

ZE syndrome (Zollinger-Ellison syndrome) This is a disease in which abnormal amounts of a hormone called gastrin are produced. This results in a vast increase in the amount of gastric acid which can cause peptic ulcers.

Index

A

Accupro 207
Accuretic 114, 207
Acepril 41
Acetoxyl 31
Achromycin 229
Acnecide 31
Acnidazil 31
Actonorm 143
Acyclovir 9
Adalat 165
Adifax 71
Adizem 78
Aerobec 28
Aerocrom 213
Aerocrom
  (with salbutamol) 215
Aerolin Autohaler 213
Alclometasone 10
Aldomet 152
Algitec 53
Alimix 55
Allegron 171
Allopurinol 11
Almodan 17
Alrheumat 131
Aludrox 143
Alvedon 177
Ambisome 18
Amiodarone 13
Amitriptyline 15
Amix 17
Amlodipine 16
Amoram 17
Amoxil 17
Amoxycillin 17
Amphocil 18
Amphotericin 18
Ampicillin 19
Ampiclox 19
Amrit 17
Anafranil 59
Angettes 21
Angiopine MR 165
Antazoline 20
Antepsin 217

Antipressan 24
Aprinox 29
Apsifen 118
Arabralene 154
Arpimycin 89
Arthrotec 74
Asmaven 213
Aspav 64, 158
Aspirin
  (acetylsalicylic acid) 21-22
Aspirin 21
Astemizole 23
Atenolol 24
Ativan 142
Atromid-S 57
Atrovent 126
Augmentin 17
Auranofin 25
Avloclor 48
Avomine 202
Axid 168
Azatadine 26
Azidothymidine 244
AZT 244

B

Bacitracin 27
Bactrim 63
Beclazone 28
Becloforte 28
Beclomethasone 28
Becodisks 28
Becotide 28
Bedranol 203
Bendrofluazide 29
Benemid 198
Benoxyl 31
Benzagel 31
Benzamycin 89
Benzocaine 30
Benzoyl peroxide 31
Benztropine 32
Benzydamine 33
Berkatens 241
Berkolol 203
Berkozide 29
Beta-adalat 165

Betahistine 34
Betaloc 154
Betamethasone 35
Beta-Prograne 203
Betim 234
Betnelan 35
Betnovate 35
Betnovate Rectal 136
BiNovum 90
BiNovum
  (with ethinyloestradiol) 169
Bioglan Hemofactor 127
Blocadren 234
Bolvidon 156
Brevinor 90
Brevinor
  (with ethinyloestradiol) 169
Bricanyl 226
Britiazim 78
Brocadopa 133
Bromazepam 36
Bromocriptine 37
Brufen 118
Buccastem 201
Budesonide 38
Bumetanide 39
Burinex 39
Buscopan 117

C

Cafergot 88
Calabren 107
Calcijex 40
Calcilat 165
Calcitriol 40
Calgel 136
Calpol 177
Calvita 127
Camcolit 139
Canesten 62
Caplenal 11
Capoten 41
Capozide 114
Caprin 21
Captopril 41
Carace 114, 138
Carace Plus 138

Norfloxacin 170
Norgeston 134
Noriday 169
Norimin 90
Noristerat 169
Normison 223
Norplant 134
Nortriptyline 171
Norval 156
Nuelin 230
Nurofen 118
Nu-seals aspirin 21
Nuvelle 134
Nycopren 159
Nystadermal 172
Nystaform 172
Nystatin 172

O

Ocusert Pilo 190
Omeprazole 173
Ondansetron 174
Opticrom 215
Optimine 26
Oramorph 158
Ortho-Novin 1/50 90
Orudis 131
Oruvail Gel 131
Oruvail 131
Otomize 69
Otosporin 115
Otrivine-Antistin 20
Ovran 90
Ovran 30
 (with ethinyloestradiol) 134
Ovranette 90
Ovranette
 (with ethinyloestradiol) 134
Ovysmen 90
Oxazepam 175
Oxprenolol 176

P

Paldesic 177
Pamergan P100 181
Pamergan P100
 (with pethidine) 202
Pameton 177
Panadol 177
Panadol Ultra 64

Panoxyl preparations 31
Paracetamol 177
Paracodol 64
Paramax 177
Paramax (paracetamol) 153
Parlodel 37
Parmid 153
Parnate 236
Parnstelin 236
Penbritin 19
Pendramine 178
Penicillamine 178
Penicillin V 186
Pentazocine 179
Pentran 188
Pepcid 93
Peptimax 53
Percutol 110
Perinal 115
Perindopril 180
Pethidine 181
Pevaryl 86
Phasal 139
Phenelzine 182
Phenergan 202
Phenindione 184
Phenoxymethylpenicillin
 (penicillin V) 186
Phentermine 187
Phenytoin 188
Phimetin 53
Physeptone 151
Pilocarpine 190
Pindolol 191
Piroxicam 192
Pizotifen 193
Plendil 94
Polyfax 27
Ponderax 95
Ponstan 148
Pravastatin 194
Prazosin 195
Predenema 196
Predfoam 196
Pred Forte 196
Prednisolone/Prednisone 196
Predsol 196
Prepulsid 55
Prestim 29, 234
Priadel 139

Primeperan 153
Primolut-N 169
Primoteston 228
Probenecid 198
Probucol 199
Procainamide 200
Procainamide Durules 200
Prochlorperazine 201
Proctofoam HC 115
Proflex 118
Proflo 164
Promethazine 202
Pronestyl 200
Propaderm 28
Propain 64, 177
Propranolol 203
Propylthiouracil 205
Proscar 96
Protamine Zinc 124
Prothiaden 83
Prozac 101
Psoradrate 81
Psorin 81
Pulmicort 38
Pyrantel 206

Q

Quellada 137
Questran 52
Quinapril 207
Quinidine 208
Quinine 209
Quinoderm
 (with hydrocortisone) 31
Quinoped 31

R

Ramipril 210
Ranitidine 211
Rastinon 235
Remedeine 177
Restandol 228
Retin-A 238
Retrovir 244
Rhinocort 38
Rhumalgen 74
Rhythmodan 80
Ridaura 25
Rimapurinol 11
Rimoxallin 17